Multidisciplinary Inte[...] for People with Diverse Needs - A Training Guide for Teachers, Students, and Professionals

Edited by:

Samuel Honório
SHERU - Sports, Health & Exercise Research Unit,
Polytechnic Institute of Castelo Branco, Portugal

Marco Batista
SHERU - Sports, Health & Exercise Research Unit,
Polytechnic Institute of Castelo Branco, Portugal

Helena Mesquita
SHERU - Sports, Health & Exercise Research Unit,
Polytechnic Institute of Castelo Branco
&
Interdisciplinary Centre of Social Sciences (CICS.NOVA), Portugal

Jaime Ribeiro
School of Health Sciences & ciTechCare - Center for Innovative
Care and Health Technology, Polytechnic of Leiria, Portugal
&
CIDTFF - Research Centre on Didactics and Technology
in the Education of Trainers, University of Aveiro, Portugal

Multidisciplinary Interventions for People with Diverse Needs -

A Training Guide for Teachers, Students, and Professionalss

Editors: Samuel Honório, Marco Batista, Helena Mesquita and Jaime Ribeiro

ISBN (Online): 978-981-14-4677-1

ISBN (Print): 978-981-14-4675-7

ISBN (Paper Back): 978-981-14-4676-4

© 2020, Bentham Books imprint.

Published by Bentham Science Publishers Pte. Ltd. Singapore. All Rights Reserved.

need for a court order if at any point you breach any terms of this License Agreement. In no event will any delay or failure by Bentham Science Publishers in enforcing your compliance with this License Agreement constitute a waiver of any of its rights.

3. You acknowledge that you have read this License Agreement, and agree to be bound by its terms and conditions. To the extent that any other terms and conditions presented on any website of Bentham Science Publishers conflict with, or are inconsistent with, the terms and conditions set out in this License Agreement, you acknowledge that the terms and conditions set out in this License Agreement shall prevail.

Bentham Science Publishers Pte. Ltd.
80 Robinson Road #02-00
Singapore 068898
Singapore
Email: subscriptions@benthamscience.net

BENTHAM SCIENCE

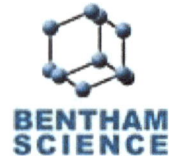

CONTENTS

FOREWORD

Multidisciplinary Interventions for People with Diverse Needs is a book written from an interdisciplinary perspective that has the objective of helping to understand the problems from people with special needs.

It is an entertaining, well written, didactic book that will be useful for students and professionals interested in studying several and different approaches related to the meaning, evaluation and intervention of the problems related to dementia, language disorders, diabetes, alterations of consciousness, celiac disease and disability in general. The different chapters offer an updated theoretical foundation that allows contextualizing and justifying the development of these issues. For the students it will be a useful work to develop the foundation and justification of research related to the final projects of degrees, master's degrees and doctoral theses.

For teachers and professionals the work will serve as a guide for teaching, for the development of the structure of training courses, for the design of evaluation models and intervention of the topics addressed in the book. The authors of this book are experts, of recognized prestige, who come mainly from the academic world, who have achieved a balance between the rigor and depth of analysis of the different topics, and the development of an accessible text for different profiles of readers and use.

Pedagogues, psychologists, students, teachers and professionals from the Social and Health Sciences, Sports Sciences, among others, will find in this book a place to lean out to discover very interesting academic, professional and human aspects related to the world of special needs.

Prof. Sixto Cubo Delgado
Universidad de Extremadura
Faculty of Education
Educational Sciences Department
Spain

PREFACE

Human diversity faces several challenges, as there are many people in situations of vulnerability due to personal and environmental factors. Vulnerable populations can experience physical, psychological, and social problems. Those include people who face great precariousness in their life and find themselves in a situation of effective vulnerability. These people need a prompt, effective and a scientific evidence-based response to overcome barriers thrown at them.

This book compiles a set of focused evidence chapters to raise awareness on the particular conditions of special populations, invoking assessment and intervention to promote better life conditions.

In the first chapter we can find an issue that affects contemporary society, the ageing population. Although living longer is an unquestionable gain, the truth is that increasing average life expectancy inevitably entails the onset of dementia, urging the need to slow its progression and minimize its impact. It presents scientifically based physical activity to combat the cognitive decline and extend the years of life with quality.

Chapter 2 raises awareness on people with brain damage with altered consciousness. The uncertainty on the patient's state of conscience leads to doubts in the course of action to follow in terms of treatment or prolongation of life. Correct assessment plays a vital role to foster best decisions and directed interventions on the patient's best interest. Situations of misdiagnosis and consequently unachieved interventions are frequent and must be improved through extended and evidence-based approaches.

People with special needs are addressed in the third chapter. We are in a global world where borders fade and anyone can pursue employment and better life outside his/her country. It may seem simple, but there are persons with constraints that cannot fulfil their needs. Not using a common language can prevent social and employment relations. Exclusion is aggravated when learning a language hampered by a functional limitation. Sensory, motor and cognitive disabilities can hinder a truthful inclusion in modern society. EN-ABILITIES is a European project that aims to enable English autonomous learning by people with diverse needs, sustained on a universal design for learning approach.

The fourth chapter focuses on the performance of activities of daily living of children with disabilities. What for many is considered acquired, for others it seems to be a difficult task. Those inattentive, may not realize the impact of having great difficulties, or not being able, to perform everyday tasks can have in the life of a child with functional limitations. Depending on others for several tasks, having reduced options for activities and encountering mobility barriers is a crucial factor for those who experience great difficulties. Knowing this and other issues can structure routines that facilitate their inclusion in the different contexts in which these children are inserted.

Autism Spectrum Disorders are discussed on the fifth chapter. It has been found that children with ASD experience difficulties processing, integrating and responding to sensory stimuli. Consequently, behaviours associated with difficulty processing and integrating sensory information create social isolation for children and their families, restrict participation in daily living activities and impact social engagement. What for some can be misbehaviour is in fact a maladaptive response to the environment and must be carefully addressed to minimize and overcome sensory processing dysfunctions. Specialized interventions such as occupational therapy using sensory integration are in order to help children with ASD respond more adequately to environmental stimuli.

Diabetes, referred in chapter six, is a modern world disease. Although it may be congenital, it also emerges from modern life style and eating habits. Aetiology aside, it can be seen that it can lead to serious problems with loss of independence and drastic reduction of quality of life. The adoption of a strategy to prevent the onset and progression of the disease are imperative. However, when it is already installed, its effects must be minimized. The combination of the intervention of different professionals seems like the procedure to adopt for an optimized approach.

Chapter seven goes through Celiac disease an increasingly visible condition, with frequent identification of more cases. The ordinary citizen is not aware of the difficulties that people suffering from this disease suffer. In catering and collective food services, mistakes that can harm a vulnerable person are frequent. It is important to raise awareness of the effects of the disease, in particular those that can make a difference in the lives of these people, avoiding things as simple as cross-contamination in food distribution, storage and handling, without ever forgetting the need for research and innovation for normalizing the diet of these people.

Animal Assisted Therapy and Developmental Disorders come to us in chapter eight. In it we can read how therapy with animals can assist in the promotion of skills, health-related issues and well-being of persons with developmental disorder. The overview presented shows the array of conditions that can benefit of this type of interventions. The basis of the intervention is the arise of a relationship that liberates the person with developmental disabilities, promoting positive emotional responses that influence neurobiological components and enhances performance in diverse areas, independent functioning, social participation and quality of life of those which are confronted with limitations due to disorders in their development.

Early in this book, physical activity was mentioned as a preventive and therapeutic intervention for people with diverse conditions. Chapter nine addresses again physical activity, but this time in people with disabilities. Due to their functional constraints, people with disabilities tend to perform less, or not to perform, physical activity that would greatly benefit them in a multidimensional way.

It reveals the need to identify the physical activity determinants in order to contribute to conceptual changes, new interventions and policies that increase the levels of physical activity on this population and, consequently, further advance in their full social inclusion.

The final chapter, chapter 10, deepens the theme of physical activity in children with disabilities. It's well known regular physical activity has a positive impact in health and lifestyle, contributing for functionality and quality of life. It is important to create opportunities for physical activity. In this context, school sports appear as a first line of intervention. Inclusion is a trend that must be completely fulfilled. Legislation protects the rights of functional diverse students and obliges to their inclusion in school activities, of which school sports cannot be an exception. Although it may seem less compelling to mandatorily engage in physical exercise, the truth is that if it is not enforced, it will probably never be performed by those who need it.

For the foregoing, this book assumes as essential when the theme are populations in situations of vulnerability. Academics, technicians, and the general population here have a source for drinking knowledge shed by scientists and based on rigorous scientific evidence.

iv

Prof. Jaime Ribeiro
School of Health Sciences & ciTechCare
Center for Innovative, Care and Health Technology
Polytechnic of Leiria
Portugal

List of Contributors

António Moreira	CIDTFF - Research Centre on Didactics and Technology in the Education of Trainers, University of Aveiro, Portugal
Andreia Inácio	School of Health Sciences & ciTechCare - Center for Innovative Care and Health Technology, Polytechnic of Leiria, Portugal
Ana Lopes	School of Health Sciences & ciTechCare - Center for Innovative Care and Health Technology, Polytechnic of Leiria, Portugal
Adilson Marques	CIPER, Faculdade de Motricidade Humana, Universidade de Lisboa, Faculdade de MotricidadeHumana, Estrada da Costa, Portugal
Bárbara Almeida	Faculdade de Motricidade Humana, UIDEF – Instituto da Educação, Universidade de Lisboa, Lisbon, Portugal
Catarina Lobão	School of Health Sciences & ciTechCare - Center for Innovative Care and Health Technology, Polytechnic of Leiria, Portugal
Danielle Blacker	Royal Hospital for Neuro-disability, London, UK
Elena Alcalde	Departament of Modern Philology, University of Alcalá, Madrid, Spain
Fernando Gomes	SpertLab, Faculdade de Motricidade Humana, Universidade de Lisboa, Lisbon, Portugal
Gladys Malafaia	Faculdade de Motricidade Humana, Universidade de Lisboa, Lisbon, Portugal
Hugo Neves	School of Health Sciences & ciTechCare - Center for Innovative Care and Health Technology, Polytechnic of Leiria, Portugal
Helena S. Reis	School of Health Sciences & ciTechCare - Center for Innovative Care and Health Technology, Polytechnic of Leiria, Portugal
Helena Mesquita	Health & Exercise Reseach Unit (SHERU, Instituto Politécnico de Castelo Branco/Centro Interdisciplinar de Ciências Sociais(CICS.NOVA)/Sport, Portugal
Inês Maldonado	Faculdade de Motricidade Humana, Universidade de Lisboa, Portugal
José Luis González	Education Faculty, University of Burgos, Spain
João Serrano	SHERU - Sports, Health and Exercise Research University, Polytechnic Institute of Castelo Branco, Portugal
Jaime Ribeiro	School of Health Sciences & ciTechCare - Center for Innovative Care and Health Technology, Polytechnic of Leiria, Portugal CIDTFF - Research Centre on Didactics and Technology in the Education of Trainers, University of Aveiro, Portugal
Liliana Teixeira	School of Health Sciences; ciTechCare - Center for Innovative Care and Health Technology, Polytechnic of Leiria & Faculdade de Medicina da Universidade de Porto, Portugal
Marco Batista	SHERU - Sports, Health and Exercise Research University, Polytechnic Institute of Castelo Branco, Portugal
Margarida Lucas	CIDTFF - Research Centre on Didactics and Technology in the Education of Trainers, University of Aveiro, Portugal

Mônica Braúna	School of Health Sciences & ciTechCare - Center for Innovative Care and Health Technology, Polytechnic of Leiria, Portugal
Miguel Peralta	CIPER, Faculdade de Motricidade Humana, Universidade de Lisboa Faculdade de MotricidadeHumana, Estrada da Costa, Portugal
Nuno Rocha	School of Health, Polytechnic Institute of Porto, Portugal
Pedro Morato	Faculdade de Motricidade Humana, UIDEF – Instituto da Educação, Universidade de Lisboa, Lisbon, Portugal
Pedro J. Bargão	School of Health Science, Polytechnic of Leiria, Portugal
Rui Gonçalves	Nursing School of Coimbra, UICISA:E - Health Sciences Research Unit: Nursing, Coimbra, Portugal
Samuel Honório	SHERU - Sports, Health and Exercise Research University, Polytechnic Institute of Castelo Branco, Portugal
Sergio Sanchez	Interfaculty Department of Evolutionary Psychology and Education, Autonomous University of Madrid, Spain
Sofia Santos	Faculdade de Motricidade Humana, UIDEF – Instituto da Educação, Universidade de Lisboa, Lisbon, Portugal
Vânia Ribeiro	School of Health Sciences & ciTechCare - Center for Innovative Care and Health Technology, Polytechnic of Leiria, Portugal
Vera Figueiredo Serafim	Faculdade de Motricidade Humana, Universidade de Lisboa, Portugal

CHAPTER 1

Exercise and Physical Activity - Contributions to Intervention in People with Dementia

Jaime Ribeiro[1,2,*]**, Marco Batista**[3]**, Samuel Honório**[3]**, João Serrano**[3] and **Helena Mesquita**[4]

[1] School of Health Sciences & ciTechCare - Center for Innovative Care and Health Technology, Polytechnic of Leiria, Portugal

[2] CIDTFF - Research Centre on Didactics and Technology in the Education of Trainers - University of Aveiro, Portugal

[3] SHERU - Sports, Health and Exercise Research Unit, Polytechnic Institute of Castelo Branco, Portugal

[4] Instituto Politécnico de Castelo Branco/Centro Interdisciplinar de Ciências Sociais (CICS.NOVA)/Sport, Health & Exercise Reseach Unit (SHERU), Portugal

Abstract: In the last few decades, the world has undergone profound demographic changes, reflected in life expectancy. We live for much longer, but we cannot say that these growing years are directly proportional to the quality of life. Dementia, in its different aetiologies, is more and more frequent with a consequent decline in the quality of life. However, cognitive decline and the onset of dementia may be delayed with the adoption of healthy lifestyle habits and therapeutic combinations that use non-pharmacological approaches such as activity and physical exercise. This chapter integrates a thorough review of the literature that characterizes ageing, cognitive decline and dementia, and it summarizes scientific evidence on the effects of physical activity on cognitive functions. Finally, recommendations are presented on the prescription of exercise for older people and elderly people with dementia. It is known that there are direct benefits (action on neurotrophic factors and neurotransmitters, among others), as well as indirect ones such as those resulting from a better vascularization of the brain. However, physical exercise requires precautions related to the conditions inherent to normal and pedagogical ageing. It is possible to perform adapted physical activity resulting from the coordination of sports and health professionals, knowledgeable of the needs and idiosyncrasies of the elderly, with cognitive decline or dementia.

Keywords: Cognitive decline, Dementia, Elderly, Physical exercise.

* **Corresponding author Jaime Ribeiro:** School of Health Sciences, Polytechnic of Leiria, Leiria, Portugal; E-mail: jaime.ribeiro@ipleiria.pt

Samuel Honório, Marco Batista, Helena Mesquita & Jaime Ribeiro (Eds.)

INTRODUCTION

This chapter summarizes the effects of physiological and pathological ageing and their cognitive implications. In the most exacerbated cases, we can observe the onset of dementia, which, despite the different aetiologies and possible evolutions, inevitably leads to deterioration of cognitive skills and, consequently, to lesser autonomy, greater dependence on caregivers and loss of quality of life.

In this way, in a multidisciplinary approach that combines Occupational Therapy and Physical Education professionals, it is important to list a set of scientific evidence that describes the benefits of exercise and physical activity in minimizing cognitive deterioration due to ageing. It also aims to submit a proposal for an exercise and physical activity program that helps seniors and their formal and informal caregivers.

Research in the area of exercise and ageing has a relatively short but very active history. There has been a major development in the research of ageing in the last two decades. Among other findings, the researchers provided evidence of potential low-cost alternative therapies for the treatment and prevention of disease and the potential to improve the quality of life, health, and overall vitality of the elderly.

The discussion about ageing-associated cognitive impairment and especially dementia is justified. In this context, we highlight Stone (2011), who stated that it is extremely rare to find an elderly person who does not have cognitive impairment. In this sense, this chapter discusses the benefits of physical activity in the ageing of the individual, in particular on one of the most frequent associated disorders - cognitive compromise.

Sustained by the scientific evidence, we want to contextualize and propose a program of exercise and physical activity as a non-pharmacological intervention for the prevention and reduction of progression of cognitive decline in individuals of advanced age.

Population ageing is a worldwide reality and in particular, in the European context where there is already an ageing index of 123.9, meaning that for every 100 young people, there are 123.9 elderly people (PORDATA, 2016).

The increase in human longevity has been a constant trend worldwide in recent decades. Improved socioeconomic conditions and nutritional resources, together with the prevention and treatment of important pathologies such as infectious, metabolic, vascular and cardiac diseases, have contributed to an increase in longevity from 60 to 80 years old during the 20th century in Western countries

(Démonet & Celsis, 2012). However, this dramatic increase in life expectancy was not accompanied by a proportional increase in quality of life for the elderly. On the contrary, generally, the increase of the life expectancy intensifies the risk of disease, deficiency, dementia and advanced ageing before the death. In the particular aspect of dementia, Santana, Farinha, Freitas, Rodrigues and Carvalho (2015) mentioned that the incidence and prevalence of dementia increase with age, doubling every five years after the sixth decade of life. They added that the estimated number of Portuguese over 60 years old and with dementia was 160287, which corresponds to 5.91% of this population. Knowing that Alzheimer's Disease represents 50-70% of the cases, there will be between 80144 and 112201 patients (Santana, Farinha, Freitas, Rodrigues & Carvalho, 2015). Kravitz, E., Schmeidler, J., & Beeri, M. S. (1990) disclosed that in the 85-year age group, more than half will have dementia and that the annual incidence rate doubles every 5 years. In 2010, Corrada, Brookmeyer, Paganini-Hill, Berlau, and Kawas already argued that the incidence of all causes of dementia is very high in people aged 90 years and older and continues to increase exponentially with age in both men and women. In this context arises the need to fight the effects of cognitive impairment and, in its more severe variant, dementia, trying to minimize its effects and delay its setting in so that individuals can live longer, but also with greater autonomy and quality of life. One of the most widely used therapies, along with vitamin supplements, used as the first line of defence against the detection of mild cognitive impairment and against the onset of dementia, is the practice of physical exercise.

However, the elderly population, because of ageing, needs special attention when delineating a program of exercise and physical activity.

AGEING - BRIEF CONTEXTUALIZATION

The current section provides a brief context for the reader to contact with the conjuncture of ageing, observing the demography and the main physiological changes, in particular, the repercussions on the brain, and the care to be taken when exercising and performing physical activity. It seeks to justify the need for the exploration of the present subject-matter in the context of contemporary society.

Sociodemography

Population ageing is a worldwide concern. There is a growing increase in the elderly population due to two main aspects: the increase in life span and the decrease in the birth rate. Human life expectancy has been increasing rapidly. Due to better health and hygiene, healthier lifestyles, enough food and better medical care, as well as the reduction of infant mortality, we can now expect to live much longer than our ancestors and in just a few generations (Brown, 2015). In this context, it is verified that the number of elderly people over 85 years of age has also been progressing, being designated as the oldest-old. The latest data revealed by The World Bank (2017)1 indicates that the number of people over 65 corresponds to 8.7% of the world population (654,567,936 people). It is noticeable the growing ageing population worldwide and it is believed that by the year 2050, the elderly will be one-fifth of the world's population and out-number children, teenagers and youth (under 10 to 24), (United Nations, 2017).

"Although the process of population ageing is most advanced in Europe and in Northern America, where more than one person in five was aged 60 or over in 2017, the populations of other regions are growing older as well. In 2050, older persons are expected to account for 35 per cent of the population in Europe, 28 percent in Northern America, 25 per cent in Latin America and the Caribbean, 24 per cent in Asia, 23 per cent in Oceania and 9 per cent in Africa." (United Nations, 2017, p.1)

Physiological Changes of Ageing

Ageing is an inescapable, progressive and irreversible process that occurs from conception until the death of the individual and is usually accompanied by a decline in the biological functions of most organs. All human systems are affected to a greater or lesser degree, and there is a global or particular decline in sensory, motor, perceptive, associative and cognitive competences. Each system begins its ageing at a given time and loses its function (or demonstrates its loss of function) at its own pace, but in a linear way (Fechine & Trompieri, 2015). It is an idiosyncratic process affecting individuals in different ways, different rhythms and different intensities. Structural and physiological changes are observed, with changes occurring at the cellular level, in the tissues, organs and systems. Inevitably, biological degradation causes problems in function. A decline in the function of an organ or system, whether due to a disturbance or to ageing itself, may affect the function of another system (Gilson, 2013). A major example is the cardiovascular system that has under its purview all the remaining organs and systems and that with ageing there is a loss of heart and blood vessel elasticity with consequent reduction of cardiac output and increase of blood pressure. The heart of an elderly person cannot accelerate as fast or pump as fast or as much blood, for example, leading to the occurrence of increased fatigue (Afiune, 2013). Although most functions may remain adequate, decreased function means that older people are less able to cope with stresses, including strenuous physical activity and exacerbated environmental changes. This decline also means that the elderly are more likely to experience side effects of physical activity. It is also known that physical stress and the environment have a greater impact on the function of some organs in particular. These organs include, as already mentioned, the heart and blood vessels, but also the urinary organs (such as the kidneys), and especially the brain.

Table **1** summarizes the main changes related to ageing which should be considered in the intervention with the elderly, in particular, in the use of exercise and physical activity.

Ageing of the Brain and Nervous System

The brain and nervous system are not different from other organs, being subjected to a higher incidence of diseases as the age progresses. Process centres of all human activities, react greatly to ageing, leading to major functional and cognitive limitations. At the neuromotor level, these limitations may translate into slower reaction speed and task performance, changes in praxis ability, poor motor coordination, poor balance and the presence of tremors. At the cognitive level, executive function impairments can be observed, for example, the subtle reduction, after the age of 70, of vocabulary, short-term memory, the ability to learn and the ability to remember words.

Table 1. Selected Physiologic Age-Related Changes.

Affected Organ or System	Physiological Changes	Clinical Manifestations
Body composition	↓ Lean body mass ↓ Muscle mass (sarcopenia) ↓ Creatinine production ↓ Skeletal mass (bone density) ↓ Total body water ↑ Percentage of adipose tissue (until age 60, then ↓until death)	Changes in drug levels (usually ↑) ↓ Strength Tendency toward dehydration
Cells	↑ DNA damage and ↓DNA repair capacity ↓ Oxidative capacity Accelerated cell senescence ↑ Fibrosis Lipofuscin accumulation	↑ Cancer risk
CNS	↓ Number of dopamine receptors ↑ Alpha-adrenergic responses ↑ Muscarinic parasympathetic responses	Tendency toward parkinsonian symptoms (*e.g.*, ↑ muscle tone, ↓ arm swing)
Ears	Loss of high-frequency hearing	↓ Ability to recognize speech
Endocrine system	↑ Insulin resistance and glucose intolerance	↑ Incidence of diabetes

(Table 1) contd.....

Affected Organ or System	Physiological Changes	Clinical Manifestations
	Menopause, ↓ estrogen and progesterone secretion ↓ Testosterone secretion ↓ Growth hormone secretion ↓ Vitamin D absorption and activation ↑ Incidence of thyroid abnormalities ↑ Bone mineral loss ↑□Secretion of ADH in response to osmolar stimuli	Vaginal dryness, dyspareunia ↓ Muscle mass ↓Bone mass ↑ Fracture risk Changes in skin Tendency toward water intoxication
Eyes	↓ Lens flexibility ↑ Time for pupillary reflexes (constriction, dilation) ↑ Incidence of cataracts	Presbyopia ↑ Glare and difficulty adjusting to changes in lighting ↓ Visual acuity
GI tract	↓ Splanchnic blood flow ↑ Transit time	Tendency toward constipation and diarrhoea
Heart	↓ Intrinsic heart rate and maximal heart rate Blunted baroreflex (less increase in heart rate in response to a decrease in BP) ↓ Diastolic relaxation ↑ Atrioventricular conduction time ↑ Atrial and ventricular ectopy	Tendency toward syncope ↓ Ejection fraction ↑ Rates of atrial fibrillation ↑ Rates of diastolic dysfunction and diastolic heart failure
Immune system	↓ T-cell function ↓ B-cell function	↑ susceptibility to infections and possibly cancer ↓ Antibody response to immunization or infection but ↑autoantibodies
Joints	Degeneration of cartilaginous tissues Fibrosis ↑ Glycosylation and cross-linking of collagen Loss of tissue elasticity	Tightening of joints Tendency toward osteoarthritis
Kidneys	↓ Renal blood flow ↓ Renal mass ↓ Glomerular filtration ↓ Renal tubular secretion and reabsorption ↓ Ability to excrete a free-water load	Changes in drug levels with ↑ risk of adverse drug effects Tendency toward dehydration
Liver	↓ Hepatic mass ↓ Hepatic blood flow ↓ Activity of the CYP 450 enzyme system	Changes in drug levels
Nose	↓ Smell	↓ Taste and consequent ↓ appetite ↑ Likelihood (slightly) of nosebleeds

(Table 1) cont.....

Affected Organ or System	Physiological Changes	Clinical Manifestations
Peripheral nervous system	↓ Baroreflex responses ↓ Beta-adrenergic responsiveness and number of receptors ↓ Signal transduction ↓ Muscarinic parasympathetic responses Preserved alpha-adrenergic responses	Tendency toward syncope ↓ Response to beta-blockers Exaggerated response to anticholinergic drugs
Pulmonary system	↓ Vital capacity ↓ Lung elasticity (compliance) ↑ Residual volume ↓FEV_1 ↑ V/Q mismatch	↑ Likelihood of shortness of breath during vigorous exercise if people are normally sedentary or if exercise is done at high altitudes ↑ Risk of death due to pneumonia ↑ Risk of serious complications (*e.g.*, respiratory failure) for patients with a pulmonary disorder
Vasculature	↓ Endothelin-dependent vasodilation ↑ Peripheral resistance	Tendency toward hypertension

↓=decreased; ↑= increased; FEV_1= forced expiratory volume in 1 sec; V/Q =ventilation/perfusion.
Source: MSD Manuals (2018)[2] Last full review/revision September 2016 by Richard W. Besdine,
Adapted from the Institute of Medicine: *Pharmacokinetics and Drug Interactions in the Elderly Workshop.*
Washington DC, National Academy Press, 1997, pp. 8–9.

It is known that ageing causes changes in brain size, brain vasculature and cognition. Cortical atrophy occurs with increasing age, as well as changes in the micro and macrostructure, from the molecular level. The incidence of stroke, white matter lesions and dementia also increases with age, moreover the impairment of memory, as well as changes in neurotransmitter and hormone levels (Peters, 2006).

The most debated neurotransmitters in relation to ageing are dopamine and serotonin. Dopamine levels decline by about 10% per decade since the onset of adulthood and have been associated with declines in cognitive and motor performance. Serotonin and levels of brain-derived neurotrophic factor also decay with advancing age and may be involved in the regulation of synaptic plasticity and neurogenesis in the adult brain. Monoamine oxidase, an important substance in the homeostasis of neurotransmitter levels, increases with age and may liberate free radicals from reactions that exceed inherent antioxidant reserves and is regarded as a significant factor in involution processes in nervous tissue (Volchegorskii *et al.*, 2004). Other factors that have been implicated in brain ageing include calcium deregulation, mitochondrial dysfunction, and the production of reactive oxygen species. Brain ageing may also suffer from altered glucose metabolism or reduced glucose or oxygen input as cerebrovascular efficiency decreases, although glucose reduction may be partly attributed to atrophy rather than any change in metabolism. Another problem commonly associated with ageing is the change in the vasculature that is associated with transient ischemic attacks, stroke and white matter lesions (Peters, 2006).

Nordon, Guimarães, Kozonoe, Mancilha and Neto (2009) presented well-known processes of cerebral ageing:

- **Cerebral atrophy with dilatation of grooves and ventricles;**

- **Loss of neurons;**

- **Granulovacuolar degeneration;**

- **Presence of neuritic plaques;**

- **Formation of Lewy bodies from alpha-synuclein;**

- **Formation of beta-amyloid plaques;**

- **Formation of neurofibrillary tangles.**

Ageing and brain consequences are inevitable, and consequently, the implications on one's activities and participation cannot be neglected.

The cortical atrophy, the decreasing amount of neurotransmitters, biochemical changes, oxidative stress and reduced blood flow are crucial aspects for the practice of physical exercise.

There are also situations in which pathological ageing may occur due to acquired lesions as sequelae of vascular accidents or dementia processes and, as already mentioned, they frequently affect the elderly, drastically reducing levels of functionality.

Cognitive Decline and Dementia

Even without an explicit diagnosis of dementia, it is generally accepted that age-related cognitive decline occurs in humans as well as in nonhuman primates (Kravitz, Schmeidler, & Beeri, 2012). The cognitive decline associated with ageing varies in terms of onset and progression, depending on factors such as education, health, personality, overall intellectual level, specific mental capacity, among others (Fechine, & Trompieri, 2015). This cognitive decline may assume different forms with lesser or greater impact on the autonomy and quality of life of the elderly, covering a broad spectrum of intensities that culminates with more serious dementia states such as Alzheimer's disease.

Dementia is the general term for a few neurological conditions, of which the main symptom includes a global decline in brain function. It is a degenerative, progressive and chronic process of the brain (Ropper & Brown, 2005), reaching different areas, resulting in different symptoms and disabilities, throughout its evolution, and uneven among people with the same pathology (Gogia & Rastogi, 2009; Sheehan, 2012; World Health Organization, 2015). It is not a disease but a collection of symptoms that result from brain damage, which are noticeable in functional changes beyond what is expected for normal ageing (World Health Organization, 2015; Gogia & Rastogi, 2009; Vreugdenhil *et al.*, 2012).

There is an impairment of at least two of the following domains: memory, language, executive functions, visuospatial ability, personality or behavioural changes (McKhann *et al.*, 2011). It can also coexist with neuropsychiatric symptoms, which are not explained by delirium or any other major psychiatric disorder, consistently associated with cognitive and / or behavioural decline.

This progressive decline in cognitive function, with greater emphasis on memory loss, deficits in some intellectual functions, behavioural and personality changes translate into loss of the notion of time and space, hamper communication, hinder relationships and quality of life and hamper a person's autonomy in performing DA's (Sheehan, 2012; Tabert *et al.*, 2002, Ngo & Holroyd-Leduc, 2015, OECD, 2017, World Health Organization, 2015; Manfrim & Schmidt, 2013).

The main dementias are Alzheimer's disease (50 to 70% of cases), frontotemporal dementia, Lewy body dementia and vascular dementia (of these, the only secondary).

By 2018, it is estimated that there are 50 million people with dementia in the world, with an economic impact of about 1 trillion Dollars (Pickett *et al.*, 2018). With the ageing of the world's population, this number is expected to rise dramatically (Kamiya, Osawa, Kondo, & Sakurai, 2018) to 66 million by 2030 and 115 million by 2050 (Vreugdenhil *et al.*, 2012; Ngo & Holroyd -Leduc, 2015). It is easily observable that it is a public health problem. According to data from the OECD, it is estimated that in 2017, 18.7 million people live with dementia in the countries belonging to that organization, which means that 1 in 69 people worldwide has dementia (OECD, 2017). Age is the main risk factor for dementia (Kamiya *et al.*, 2018), increasing its prevalence rate as age progresses (Demaerschalk, Woodruff, & Caselli, 2007; Fedor, Garcia, & Gunstad, 2015; Santana, Farinha, Freitas, Rodrigues, & Carvalho, 2015). According to data from the OECD (2017), the dementia prevalence rate for people over 90 years of age residing in the OECD countries is 41%, from 2% between 65 and 69, from 4% between 70 and 74 years, 7% between 75 and 79, 12% between 80 and 84, and

20% between 85 and 89.

After a light approach to the diversity of the aetiology of the cognitive decline due to the progression of age, it is interesting to summarize that physical exercise often appears as frontline therapy. Martelli (2013), in his literature review paper, listed cognitive stimulation programs, reality-oriented psychotherapy, occupational therapy, group activities, caregiver training, and other procedures, such as regular physical activity, which have provided beneficial impact for attenuation of cognitive decline and improvement of behavioural disorders in patients with AD.

NEUROPROTECTIVE AND REHABILITATIVE EFFECT OF EXERCISE ON COGNITIVE FUNCTIONS

There is accumulated evidence that exercise brings profound benefits to brain functioning (Van Pragg, 2009). Extensive research in humans suggests that exercise may have benefits to overall health and cognitive function, particularly in adult life, improving cognitive functions and lowers the risk for age-related cognitive decline (Winter, *et al*., 2009). Still, there are authors who advanced the findings that there is a link between physical activity/exercise and improved cognitive functioning and reduced risk of dementia (Brown, Pfeiffer & Martins, 2013).

There is a consensus that there are protective factors that reduce cardiovascular risks such as regular exercise, a healthy diet and low to moderate alcohol intake, which seem to aid brain ageing, as does increased cognitive effort in the course of education or professional activity.

There are several randomized control trials on the benefits of exercise for those who have Alzheimer's disease. It is therefore pertinent to emphasize that physical inactivity is a modifiable risk factor, which accelerates cognitive decline in the elderly (Fedor *et al*., 2015).

Although there are several studies on physical exercise for people with Alzheimer's disease, it is difficult to make comparisons between them. However, it has been observed that in longer interventions with higher intensities, the patients show better results (Fedor *et al*., 2015). However, recently, research has emerged indicating that prolonged intervention is not necessary to achieve positive results (Fedor *et al*., 2015).

In one study, the effects of an aerobic exercise program versus a non-aerobic stretching and toning (control) program were evaluated for 26 weeks (6 months) relative to memory, executive functions, functional capacity and depression in people in an early stage of Alzheimer's disease.

It has been found that aerobic exercise in these individuals is associated with functional capacity benefits and that improvements in cardiorespiratory fitness lead to improvements in memory and changes in brain volume, that is, reduction in hippocampal atrophy (Morris *et al.*, 2017).

In cognitive terms, physical exercise improves several aspects such as cognition in globality, attention, executive functions and memory (Fedor *et al.*, 2015).

Daily exercise programs and daily walks under the supervision of the caregiver show positive impacts on the physical and cognitive function, as well as on the level of independence in ADL (Vreugdenhil *et al.*, 2012).

It is also known that physical activity induces several neurotransmitters, including serotonin, acetylcholine, dopamine, epinephrine and norepinephrine (Sutoo & Akiyama, 2003). Winter and colleagues (2007) advanced that peripheral levels of catecholamines (dopamine, epinephrine and norepinephrine) increase in humans immediately after exercise. Similarly, it was found that exercise can change cortical activity due to the increase of activity of receptor neurotransmitter subtypes (Sarbadhikari & Saha, 2006).

Voluntary exercise induces the expression of genes associated with plasticity, increasing levels of brain-derived neurotrophic factor (BDNF), as well as other growth factors, in addition to promoting cerebral vascularization, neurogenesis, functional neuronal structure and neuronal resistance to injury. Significantly, these effects occur in the hippocampus, a central brain region for learning and memory (Cotman & Berchtold 2002).

Phillips, Baktir, Srivatsan, and Salehi (2014) developed a review paper that exposed that sustained exercise plays a role in modulating anti-inflammatory effects and may play a role in preserving cognitive function in ageing and neuropathological conditions. They reinforce that recent evidence suggests that myokines released by muscle exercise affect the expression of brain-derived neurotrophic factor synthesis in the dentate gyrus of the hippocampus, justifying the improvement of cognitive conditions in adults suffering from neurodegenerative conditions.

Kravitz, Schmeidler and Beeri (2012) also equated the influence of physical exercise on plasticity and brain reserves but highlighted the effect on the reduction of risk factors for dementia such as diabetes, other metabolic conditions and cardiovascular diseases.

The research conducted by Arcoverde *et al.* (2008) with 37 elderly patients with AD and that of Petroianu, Capanema, Silva and Braga (2010) with 393 elderly individuals over 80 years of age determined that the association of physical activity with cognitive exercises slows the decline in cognitive functions, reducing the risk of dementia.

Nicola (2009), and Eric *et al.* (2011) suggested an attenuating effect of exercise not only on brain ageing but also on atherosclerotic cerebrovascular diseases. Ahlskog (2011) conducted a meta-analysis using the terms cognition and exercise (in Pubmed and others) to verify whether physical exercise as a therapeutic strategy favours the preventive or modifying treatment of dementia and brain ageing. It was found that exercise should not be neglected as an important therapeutic strategy, observing evidence of the neuroprotective effect of exercise on cognition and attenuation of cognitive decline, namely: reduced risk of dementia associated with exercise in middle age; better cognitive scores after 6 to 12 months of exercise among patients with dementia or mild cognitive impairment; improvement in cognitive scores through aerobic exercise in healthy adults; aerobic exercise in the elderly was associated with significantly higher volumes of the hippocampus and better spatial memory; aerobic exercise attenuates age-related volume loss of gray matter. Cross-sectional studies reported significantly higher volumes in the hippocampus or gray matter among physically active elderly as compared to sedentary elderly. The cognitive networks of the brain studied with functional magnetic resonance showed improved connectivity after 6 to 12 months of physical exercise. Animal studies indicate that exercise facilitates neuroplasticity through a variety of biomechanisms, with better results, and the induction of brain neurotrophic factors by exercise has also been confirmed with evidence in multiple animal studies with evidence for this process in humans.

Philips (2014) undertook a review study to verify the neuroprotective effects of physical activity on the brain, particularly trophic factor signalling. A total of 140 articles dating from 1991 to 2014 were studied, suggesting that physical activity is an effective means to improve cognitive function at all ages, particularly in the elderly who are more vulnerable to neurodegenerative disorders. In addition to improving cardiac and immune performance, physical activity alters the production of trophic factor and, in turn, function and structure in critical areas for cognition. Sustained exercise plays a role in modulating the anti-inflammatory effects and may play a role in preserving cognitive function in ageing and in neuropathological conditions. In addition, there is evidence to suggest that myokines released during exercise by muscles affect the expression of neurotrophic factor synthesis in the dentate gyrus of the hippocampus, a finding that may lead to the identification of new and important therapeutic mediating factors, considering the increasing number of individuals with cognitive disabilities worldwide.

As can be observed from the foregoing, the literature suggests that exercise may have favourable effects on brain neuroplasticity and resilience in brain ageing and counteract neurodegeneration. Understanding how these factors contribute to cognition is imperative and is an important first step in developing non-pharmacological therapeutic strategies to improve cognition in vulnerable populations.

Within this logic, a set of prescriptive exercise principles has been identified (Table **2**), according to several authors, in order to standardize an approach to the elderly with and at risk of cognitive impairment.

From the above, it is readily apparent that in order to discuss the benefits of exercise for older adults, it is important to understand the various rehabilitation outcomes that exercise can influence. These include medical outcomes such as morbidity and mortality, cognitive outcomes, functional and disability outcomes and psycho-behavioural outcomes.

CONSIDERATIONS IN THE PRESCRIPTION OF PHYSICAL EXERCISE

Given the inherent conditioning factors of ageing, and in particular, in cases where there is associated pathology, an interprofessional approach between health and physical activity professionals, as in this chapter, becomes extremely important.

In the elderly, consideration should be given to the presence of concomitant noncardiac diseases, such as those on the pulmonary, cardiovascular, osteoarticular or neurological systems, which limit functional status and may impair adequate cardiovascular evaluation during exercise (Wellington *et al.*, 2013). This age group requires a careful study of comorbidities that, at the very least, can interfere directly with exercise modality and intensity, such as atherosclerosis, hypertension, reduction of bone density, osteoarticular problems and motor control. Due to these changes, the elderly must obtain clinical approval before starting an exercise routine, especially if they were previously sedentary or suffering from chronic illness.

Furthermore, dehydration should be seriously considered by the frequency that occurs in these individuals, even without exercise, with the inherent clinical consequences, but also with the occurrence of increased fatigue, dizziness and vertigo, and in more severe cases, irritability and confusion. When practicing exercise, it is especially important to ensure the adequate intake of liquids as for any other individual, with the particularity that the elderly dehydrate by the less thirst sensation caused by less sensorial input. The reduction of cardiovascular and cardiopulmonary reflexes in response to hypovolaemia, elevated plasma concentrations of atrial natriuretic peptide and Renin-angiotensin depression in the elderly, as well as reduced cingulate cortex activity may influence thirst mechanisms in elderly individuals (McKinley, 2009). 1.5L to 2L of water per day should be ingested to avoid dehydration and avoid exercise during extreme temperatures.

Table **3** presents a summary of the exercise recommendations for older adults written by Frankel, Bean and Frontera (2006) and illustrates clearly the contraindications to the development of physical activity with the elderly. It addresses the most frequently developed modes in exercise programs: Strength, endurance, balance, and flexibility.

Table 2. Prescriptive reference data for the elderly with dementia.

Authors	Objective	Sample	Intensity	Frequency	Results	Exercises
Yan, S. and colleagues. (2008):	To verify the effect of exercise on elderly demented women.	30 women (15 EG e 15 CG).	30 to 60% of max VO$_2$	30 to 60 min per session between 2 to 3 times per week.	The results suggest that aerobic exercise is associated with a reduced risk of cognitive impairment and dementia and may delay the disease. A convincing argument is seen by two plausible biological paths. First, a convergence of evidence from studies suggesting that aerobic exercise may attenuate the progression of neurodegenerative processes and changes in the loss of synapses, and directly influence the facilitation of neuroprotective neurotrophic factors and neuroplasticity. Second is the cerebrovascular disease. Cerebrovascular load contributes to the risk of dementia, especially through small vessel disease. Vascular risk factors are well known for the reduction of aerobic exercise. Therefore, moderate-intensity physical exercise should be considered as a prescription to decrease cognitive risks and decrease cognitive decline across the age spectrum.	

(Table 2) cont.....

Authors	Objective	Sample	Intensity	Frequency	Results	Exercises
Groppo, H. and col. (2012).	To analyse the effects of a physical activity program on depressive symptoms and quality of life of elderly people with Alzheimer's Disease.	12 (6 EG and 6 CG)	60 to 80% of MHR	3 non-consecutive days per week for 24 months.	Currently, the practise of regular physical activity is seen as a benefit, since the depressive patient involved with this practice may result in positive feedback from others, increasing their self-esteem. The act of exercising can serve as a distraction from negative thoughts and mastery of new habits may be important. The social contact provided by the context of the practice of physical activity can be an important mechanism, as physical activity causes physiological effects such as changes in the concentration of endorphins and monoamines, which can act beneficially on depression, decreasing anxiety, tension and stress.	
Eric, A. and col. (2009)	Exercise as a preventive and alternative factor in the treatment of elderly people with dementia.	29 elderly	60% of MHR	3 days a week, 20 to 30 minutes per session	The research demonstrates that exercise improves subjective and objective light cognitive functions in older adults. The benefits of physical activity were evident after 6 months and were maintained for another 12 months. After the intervention was interrupted, the mean improvement of 0.69 points in ADAS-Cog as compared to the control group during the 18 months was tenuous but very important considering the modest amount of physical activity applied to the study participants.	
Nicola, T and col. (2009)	Relate the effect of physical exercise on Cognitive Function of elderly at risk of Alzheimer's Disease.	60	Low to moderate	150 minutes per week (3 sessions of 50 min)	Exercise was associated with statistically positive results in the treatment of elderly patients with dementia. The meta-analysis results suggest a major treatment effect for health-related physical fitness components, and a global average treatment effect for physical, cognitive, functional, and behavioural changes. Preliminary results show the efficacy of exercises for people with dementia and cognitive problems.	Aerobic exercise; strength training; gymnastic circuit.

(Table 2) cont.....

Authors	Objective	Sample	Intensity	Frequency	Results	Exercises
Heyn, P and col. (2004).	To verify the effects of physical exercise in the elderly with cognitive impairment and dementia.	2020	Low 60% to 80% MHR	3-week sessions, non-consecutive days, a total of 24 weeks	The provision of physical activity is an accessible and effective method to improve cognitive functions at all ages, particularly the elderly who are more vulnerable and have neurodegenerative disorders. The chronic effects of physical activity on inflammatory processes, particularly in individuals with an underlying inflammatory condition, should be better understood in such a way that the nature of the physical activity and its inducing health benefits can be harnessed in vulnerable populations. A further refinement of the mechanisms by which myokines are released by the peripheral muscles during exercise is understood by the synthesis mechanisms of BDNF that may lead to the identification of new therapeutically important factors and that measure these effects. Moreover, since most of the synthesis of BDNF occurs in the hippocampus, there may be new technologies developed in the future to quantify the release of BDNF from the brain rather than in total circulation. The availability of new nanotechnology systems and methods for collecting blood samples locally at the cellular level may help deepen the understanding of the type of intensity of physical activity that induces BDNF synthesis in the brain.	Functional ability (agility, balance, strength endurance and aerobic capacity) Cognitive tasks (countdown, recognition of shapes, colours, tasks of verbal fluency).
Cristy, P. and col. (2014).	To analyse the neuroprotective effect of physical activity in cerebral terms.	78 elderly	low	3 to 6 times a week, 45 minutes for 23 weeks	Physical activity offers an accessible and effective method to improve cognitive function at all ages, particularly the elderly who are most vulnerable to neurodegenerative disorders.	Stationary bike, basic motor skills circuit.

(Table 2) cont.....

Authors	Objective	Sample	Intensity	Frequency	Results	Exercises
Li Wang, M and col. (2006).	To determine if the physical function is associated with the incidence of dementia Alzheimer's disease	2288 people 65 years of age and older without dementia participated. Individuals were registered from 1994 to 1996 and followed up until October 2003.		Participants who exercised at least 3 times a week were classified as regular practitioners	Lower levels of physical performance were associated with an increased risk of dementia and Alzheimer's disease. The study suggests that poor physical function predicts the onset of dementia and Alzheimer's disease and that higher levels of physical activity appear to be associated with a later onset of pathology.	Physical exercise was assessed by asking participants how many days each week they performed each of the following exercises for at least 15 minutes at a time during the last year: walking, cycling, aerobics or callisthenics, swimming, water aerobics, bodybuilding or stretching and other exercises.
Rolland, Y. and col. (2007)	To investigate the efficacy of exercise to improve the ability to perform activities of daily living, physical performance and nutrition in decreasing the state of behavioural disorder and depression in patients with Alzheimer's disease	A total of 134 patients with ambulatory capacity with mild to severe Alzheimer's disease participated.		Twice a week of walking, strength, balance and flexibility	A simple exercise program, 1 hour twice a week, has led to a significantly slower decline in behavioural disorders and depression in Alzheimer's patients living in nursing homes as compared to those who only maintain the routine of medical care.	Program of collective exercises with a duration of 1 hour, or routine of medical care for 12 months.
Etgen, T., and col. (2010) N.I	Examine whether physical activity is associated with incidents of cognitive impairment.	3903 participants, aged 55 and over, were enrolled between 2001 and 2003 and followed for 2 years.		Practice physical activity such as walking, cycling, swimming, gardening or climbing stairs or other exercises. (Classified as no activity, moderate activity [3 times / week] and high activity [3 times / week])	Moderate or high physical activity is associated with a reduced incidence of cognitive impairment over two years of follow-up.	

(Table 2) cont.....

Authors	Objective	Sample	Intensity	Frequency	Results	Exercises
Vercambre, M. and col. (2011)	To assess whether individuals with vascular disease or risk factors have substantially higher rates of cognitive decline.	A total of 2809 women 65 years of age or older, with a prevalence of at least three coronary risk factors. Recreational physical activity was assessed at the baseline (October 1995 to June 1996) and every 2 years between December 1998 and July 2000.	Accelerated pace. Standard rhythm of walking (3.2 km/h[easy rhythm], 3.2-4.7 km/h[normal rhythm], 4.8-6.3 km /h [accelerated rhythm], or 6.4 km/h[very fast rate]). Quantification of values and MET in function of the registered activities, with Cumulative of 30 minutes daily.	Equivalent to daily walks. hiking, jogging, running, tennis, squash, swimming, machines; Aerobic exercise, aerobic dance. And lower intensity exercise, including yoga, stretching or toning. Climbing flights of stairs.	Regular physical activity, including gait, has been associated with better preservation of cognition in elderly women with vascular disease or with risk factors. Walking regularly is strongly related to slower rates of cognitive decline, exerting a greater prophylactic factor in younger women.	
Sink, K. and col. (2015)	To determine whether a 24-month physical activity program results in improved cognitive function, reduced risk of mild cognitive impairment or dementia, or both.	Participants were 1635 American adults from February 2010 to December 2011. Participants were sedentary adults aged 70-89 who were at risk of mobility impairment but able to walk 400 m.	The physical activity sessions progressed toward a goal of 30 minutes of walking at moderate intensity, 10 minutes of primarily lower-extremity strength training with ankle weights, and 10 minutes of balance training and large muscle group flexibility exercises.	Three to four times a week of walking, strength, flexibility and balance training.	Among sedentary elderly, this 24-month study based on a moderate-intensity physical activity program as compared to a health education program did not result in improvements in overall or specific cognitive function.	
Toots, A. e col. (2016)	To investigate the effects of a high-intensity functional exercise program on independence in activities of daily living (DLA) and balance in the elderly with dementia and whether the effects of exercise differed between types of dementia.	Participants were 186 Swedish individuals aged 65 years or over with dementia. Experimental group of 93 participants and 93 participants in a control group.		Program of high-intensity functional exercises, balance exercises and limb strength in 5 weekly exercise sessions, with four to seven months of intervention in 45-minute sessions.	Positive effect on exercise interaction with dementia groups. In older adults institutionalized with mild to moderate dementia, a program of high-intensity functional exercises seems to slow the decline in DAL independence and improve balance, although only in participants with non-Alzheimer's dementia.	

(Table 2) cont.....

Authors	Objective	Sample	Intensity	Frequency	Results	Exercises
Suo, C (2016)	To examine through MRI, structural, functional and spontaneous changes in the brain, centred in the hippocampus and posterior cingulate regions, therapeutically relevant triggered by exercise and/or cognitive program.	Participants included 100 Australian elderly individuals (68 women, mean age = 70.1, ± 6.7, 55-87 years) with mild dementia and cognitive impairment.	Resistance: Intensity, 3 sets of 8 repetitions of every 5-6 exercises/session for most major muscle groups (chest press, leg press, sitting row, abduction, knee extension). Stretching: Seated, designed not to increase the aerobic frequency or improve balance or strength.	Hydraulic resistance machines for strength training. Sitting stretching. Mean weekly sessions were 2.3 or 44.6 sessions in absolute value, in the trial period, for a total of 26 weeks, for 90 minutes per session.	The connectivity between the hippocampus and the frontal cortex was superior. The results indicate that physical and cognitive training depends on discrete neuronal mechanisms for its therapeutic efficacy, information that may help to develop preventive strategies.	

Table 3. Synthesis of exercise recommendations for older adult patients (Translated and adapted from Frankel, Bean & Frontera, 2006, p.240).

Mode	Benefits	Precautions
Strength	Improve daily function Reduce disability Reduce blood pressure Reduce Arthritis Pain Increase aerobic capacity in congestive heart failure	Monitor vital signs in patients with known coronary artery disease, pulmonary dysfunction. Monitor fatigue in patients with neurological injuries. Initiate with reduced weight in subjects with unstable osteoarthritis (OA) of the knee.
Resistance	Reduce blood pressure Improve lipid profiles Lower cardiac mortality Improve insulin sensitivity Improve lung disease symptoms and reduce associated disability Reduce stroke-associated weakness and improve energy expenditure Reduce pain and improve function in OA and rheumatoid arthritis	Monitor O_2 saturation in patients with lung disease and use supplemental oxygen when necessary. Monitor vital signs in patients with heart and lung failure. Individuals with vascular claudication should exercise only below the point of pain. Monitor patients with neurological deficits for fatigue, and schedule exercise and rest accordingly.
Balance	Reduced risk of falls Improvement of the strength of the lower limbs Improved functionality	Control the pain where necessary. Prescribe the appropriate auxiliary devices in an adjunctive manner. Consider evaluation of bone mineral density when appropriate; Supplement of vitamin D and calcium.
Flexibility	Little studied Conclusive recommendations on flexibility training and functional outcomes for older adults remain unfounded (Stathokostas, Little, Vandervoort, & Paterson, 2012)	No clear contraindications Begin with gentle stretching, supervised orthopaedic injuries. Observe osteoarticular pathology.

Given the evidence presented, we propose the following exercise program (Table 4) as prophylactic action against cognitive impairment. Fundamentally, the objective is to maintain the independence and autonomy of individuals, as well as an active and continuous participation.

Table 4. Proposed prescriptive program as a preventive form (Adapted from Rimmer, 2003).

Training	Frequency	Duration	Intensity	Progression
Warm-up and a return to calm (Walking and mobilization)	Before and after each session	5 – 10 min	Low	
Aerobic (hiking, biking, water walking, swimming)	5 days / week	10 min per session	Low	Increase 10 to 15 min per day for 5 to 7 weeks
Strength (Supine, extension of triceps, biceps curls, squatting, arm flexing on the wall or chair)	3 days/week	1 set of 10 to 12 repetitions	Elastics and/or complete all exercises in 10 to 15 min	If necessary, start sitting. Evolve in bipedal posture according to limiting ability. Increase to 3 sets of 12 repetitions in 3 to 6 weeks.
Flexibility (All major muscle groups)	5 days/week	3-5 repetitions; Maintain for 10 - 30 sec	Movements within range without pain	
Neuro-muscular (Walk, balance and coordination circuits)	5 days/week	5-10 minutes 1 series of 3 repetitions of 1 balance circuit and 1 coordination	Within the individual's capacity without exceeding 80% MHR	Evolve to 3 sets of 3 repetitions of 1 balance circuit and 1 coordination

Adapted from Rimmer (2003).

As a summary, it can be said that for older adults, three to five days of moderate-intensity activities such as walking and/or swimming, or even cycling, are recommended for between 30 and 60 minutes per week sessions of 10 to 15 minutes. Depending on the physical and cognitive abilities of the individual (security protection), these activities can be carried out outdoors or indoors, with the use of treadmills or different types of cycle ergometers that allow to perform the activity sitting in chairs or using the upper limbs. Each exercise session should have at least five minutes of slow activity. In order to increase resistance in strength training, the elderly should use light weights or even elastic bands in order to perform between 8 and 10 repetitions.

From what has been read so far, it is observed that the elderly are a particular population due to the associated physical and psychological conditions. The preventive or therapeutic approach will always be considered in a biopsychosocial way, not neglecting the cognitive impairment that may have already been established, as well as the psychological and motivational component of the elderly and their caregivers. Other considerations that may aid the promotion of physical activity by an elderly individual include:

- Ensuring that exercise programs reflect the preferences of the elderly;
- Encouraging the elderly to attend physical activity sessions at least once or twice a week, explaining the benefits of regular physical activity;
- Advising older people and their caregivers on how to exercise safely. Provide useful examples of activities in daily life that would help achieve this (*e.g.* shopping, housework, gardening, cycling).
- Encouraging regular feedback from participants and use it to inform about the program and to measure levels of motivation.
- In collaboration with older people and their caregivers, offering a variety of low to moderate intensity walking, swimming and cycling schemes with a customized choice of contexts to suit different competencies and preferences.

CONCLUDING REMARKS

The growing research on the preventive benefits of exercise for health in the elderly has been generated by the growing percentage of this population. Some data are preliminary, but many important conclusions can be drawn that indicate benefits for the care and functional capacity of the elderly.

The prescription of vitamin supplements and physical exercise is already frequent for those who show signs of cognitive decline. Different studies have identified physiological benefits to the cognitive ability of the elderly due to the practice of physical activity.

However, physical exercise is often what the elderly cannot do. Musculoskeletal and cardiovascular changes due to ageing, risk of falls, motor slowing and reduction of protective reflexes are just a few of the many situations that affect the elderly, which should be considered when prescribing physical activity.

The exercise should be advised through an interprofessional team that brings together the specific knowledge of sports and health professionals such as Occupational Therapists, in order to adapt activity and physical exercise, improve safety and maximize effects.

NOTES

[1] Available from: https://data.worldbank.org/ indicator/SP.POP.65UP.TO?end= 2017&start=1960&view=chart

[2] Accessed on December 16th, 2018, from: https://www.msdmanuals.com/profes-sional/geriatrics/approach-to-the-geriatric-patient/physical-changes-with-aging

CONSENT FOR PUBLICATION

Not applicable.

CONFLICT OF INTEREST

The author confirms that this chapter contents have no conflict of interest.

ACKNOWLEDGEMENTS

Declared none.

REFERENCES

Afiune, A. (2013). Envelhecimento Cardiovascular. In: Freitas, E., Py, L., Cançado, F. , Doll, J., & Gorzoni, M. (Eds). *Tratado de Geriatria e Gerontologia*, Riode Janeiro: Guanabara Koogan. (pp. 557-565).

Ahlskog, J.E., Geda, Y.E., Graff-Radford, N.R., Petersen, R.C. (2011). Physical exercise as a preventive or disease-modifying treatment of dementia and brain aging. *Mayo Clin. Proc., 86*(9), 876-884.
[http://dx.doi.org/10.4065/mcp.2011.0252] [PMID: 21878600]

Alzheimer Portugal (AP). (2017). *Défice Cognitivo Ligeiro.* Retrieved 11/01/2017 from: http://alzheimerportugal.org/pt/defice-cognitivo-ligeiro

Arcoverde, C., Deslandes, A., Rangel, A., Rangel, A., Pavão, R., Nigri, F., Engelhardt, E., Laks, J. (2008). Role of physical activity on the maintenance of cognition and activities of daily living in elderly with Alzheimer's disease. *Arq. Neuropsiquiatr., 66*(2B), 323-327.
[http://dx.doi.org/10.1590/S0004-282X2008000300007] [PMID: 18641864]

Besdine, R. (2017). Physical changes with aging *MSD Manual: professional version.* Retrieved 16/12/2018 from: https://www.msdmanuals.com/professional/geriatrics/approach-to-the-geriatric-patient/physical-changes-with-aging

Brown, B.M., Peiffer, J.J., Martins, R.N. (2013). Multiple effects of physical activity on molecular and cognitive signs of brain aging: can exercise slow neurodegeneration and delay Alzheimer's disease? *Mol. Psychiatry, 18*(8), 864-874.
[http://dx.doi.org/10.1038/mp.2012.162] [PMID: 23164816]

Brown, G.C. (2015). Living too long: the current focus of medical research on increasing the quantity, rather than the quality, of life is damaging our health and harming the economy. *EMBO Rep., 16*(2), 137-141.
[http://dx.doi.org/10.15252/embr.201439518] [PMID: 25525070]

Corrada, M.M., Brookmeyer, R., Paganini-Hill, A., Berlau, D., Kawas, C.H. (2010). Dementia incidence continues to increase with age in the oldest old: the 90+ study. *Ann. Neurol., 67*(1), 114-121.
[http://dx.doi.org/10.1002/ana.21915] [PMID: 20186856]

Cotman, C.W., Berchtold, N.C. (2002). Exercise: a behavioral intervention to enhance brain health and

plasticity. *Trends Neurosci., 25*(6), 295-301.
[http://dx.doi.org/10.1016/S0166-2236(02)02143-4] [PMID: 12086747]

Phillips, C., Baktir, M.A., Srivatsan, M., Salehi, A. (2014). Neuroprotective effects of physical activity on the brain: a closer look at trophic factor signaling. *Front. Cell. Neurosci., 8*, 170. [Stony Brook, USA.].
[http://dx.doi.org/10.3389/fncel.2014.00170] [PMID: 24999318]

Démonet, J-F., Celsis, P. (2012). *Ageing of the Brain, in Pathy's Principles and Practice of Geriatric Medicine.* (5ᵗʰ ed., Vol. 1 & 2). Chichester: John Wiley & Sons, Ltd..

Eric, A., Yonas,, , Geda, E., Neill, R., Ronald, C. (2011). Physical Exercise as a Preventive or Disease-Modifying Treatment of Dementia and Brain Aging. *Mayo Clinic Proocedings* (Vol. 86, pp. 876-884). USA.

Etgen, T., Sander, D., Huntgeburth, U., Poppert, H., Förstl, H., Bickel, H. (2010). Physical activity and incident cognitive impairment in elderly persons: the INVADE study. *Arch. Intern. Med., 170*(2), 186-193.
[http://dx.doi.org/10.1001/archinternmed.2009.498] [PMID: 20101014]

Fechine, B. R. A., Trompieri, N. (2015). O processo de envelhecimento: as principais alterações que acontecem com o idoso com o passar dos anos. *InterSciencePlace. 1*(20).

Fedor, A., Garcia, S., Gunstad, J. (2015). The effects of a brief, water-based exercise intervention on cognitive function in older adults. *Arch. Clin. Neuropsychol., 30*(2), 139-147.
[http://dx.doi.org/10.1093/arclin/acv001] [PMID: 25638041]

Frankel, J.E., Bean, J.F., Frontera, W.R. (2006). Exercise in the elderly: research and clinical practice. *Clin. Geriatr. Med., 22*(2), 239-256, vii.
[http://dx.doi.org/10.1016/j.cger.2005.12.002] [PMID: 16627076]

Freitas, E., Py, L., Neri, A., Cançado, F., Doll, J., Gorzoni, M. (2013). *Tratado de geriatria e gerontologia.* (pp. 262-276). Rio de Janeiro: Guanabara Koogan.

Gilson, L. (2013). Mecanismos Biológicos do Envelhecimento. In: Freitas, E., Py, L., Neri, A., Cançado, F., Doll, J., & Gorzoni, M. (Eds.). *Tratado de geriatria e gerontologia.* Rio de Janeiro: Guanabara Koogan. (pp. 76-101).

Gogia, P.P., Rastogi, N. (2009). *Clinical Alzheimer Rehabilitation.* New York: Springer Publishing Company.

Groppo, H., Nascimento, C., Stella, F., Gobbi, S., Oliani, M. (2012). Efeitos de um programa de atividade física sobre os sintomas depressivos e a qualidade de vida de idosos com demência de Alzheimer. *Rev. Bras. Educ. Fís. Esporte, 26*(4), 543-551. [out./dez. São Paulo, Brasil.].
[http://dx.doi.org/10.1590/S1807-55092012000400002]

Heyn, P., Abreu, B.C., Ottenbacher, K.J. (2004). The effects of exercise training on elderly persons with cognitive impairment and dementia: a meta-analysis. *Arch. Phys. Med. Rehabil., 85*(10), 1694-1704.
[http://dx.doi.org/10.1016/j.apmr.2004.03.019] [PMID: 15468033]

Instituto Nacional de estatística *Dia Mundial da População.* Retrieved 11/01/2017. From: https://www.ine.pt/xportal/xmain?xpid=INE&xpgid=ine_destaques&DESTAQUESdest_boui=224679354& DESTAQUESmodo=2&xlang=pt

Kravitz, E., Schmeidler, J., Beeri, M.S. (2012). Cognitive decline and dementia in the oldest-old. *Rambam Maimonides Med. J., 3*(4), e0026.
[http://dx.doi.org/10.5041/RMMJ.10092] [PMID: 23908850]

Kwak, Y.S., Um, S.Y., Son, T.G., Kim, D.J. (2008). Effect of regular exercise on senile dementia patients. *Int. J. Sports Med., 29*(6), 471-474.
[http://dx.doi.org/10.1055/s-2007-964853] [PMID: 18050054]

Lautenschlager, N.T., Cox, K.L., Flicker, L., Foster, J.K., Van Bockxmeer, F.M., Xiao, J., Greenop, K. R., & Almeida, O.P. (2008). Effect of physical activity on cognitive function in older adults at risk for Alzheimer disease: a randomized trial. *JAMA*, 300(9), 1027-1037. [https://doi.org/10.1001/jama.300.9.1027][PMID: 18768414]

Li, R., Yu, L. (2016). Physical activity and prevention of Alzheimer's disease. *J. Sport Health Sci., 5*(4), 381-382. [China].
[http://dx.doi.org/10.1016/j.jshs.2016.10.008] [PMID: 29067218]

Manfrim, A. & Schimdt, (2013). Diagnóstico diferencial das demências. In Freitas, E., Py, L., Cançado, F. , Doll, J., & Gorzoni, M. (Eds). *Tratado de geriatria e gerontologia*. Rio de Janeiro: Guanarabara Koogan, Pp. 262-276.

Martelli, A. (2013). Alterações Cerebrais e os Efeitos do Exercício Físico no Melhoramento Cognitivo dos Portadores da Doença de Alzheimer. *Saúde e Desenvolvimento Humano, 1*(1), 49.

McKhann, G.M., Knopman, D.S., Chertkow, H., Hyman, B.T., Jack, C.R., Jr, Kawas, C.H., Klunk, W.E., Koroshetz, W.J., Manly, J.J., Mayeux, R., Mohs, R.C., Morris, J.C., Rossor, M.N., Scheltens, P., Carrillo, M.C., Thies, B., Weintraub, S., Phelps, C.H. (2011). The diagnosis of dementia due to Alzheimer's disease: recommendations from the National Institute on Aging-Alzheimer's Association workgroups on diagnostic guidelines for Alzheimer's disease. *Alzheimers Dement., 7*(3), 263-269.
[http://dx.doi.org/10.1016/j.jalz.2011.03.005] [PMID: 21514250]

McKinley, M. (2009). Thirst. *Handbook of Neuroscience for the Behavioral Sciences.* (Vol. 2, pp. 680-709). Hoboken, NJ: John Wiley and Sons.
[http://dx.doi.org/10.1002/9780470478509.neubb002035]

Morris, J. K., Vidoni, E. D., Johnson, D. K., Van Sciver, A., Mahnken, J. D., Honea, R. A., & Burns, J. M. (2017). Aerobic exercise for Alzheimer's disease: a randomized controlled pilot trial. *PloS one*, 12(2). Pp. 1-14. [https://doi.org/10.1371/journal.pone.0170547] [PMID: 28187125]

Netto, M. (2002). *Gerontologia: A velhice e o envelhecimento em visão globalizada..* São Paulo: Editora Atheneu.

Ngo, J., & Holroyd-Leduc, J. M. (2014). Systematic review of recent dementia practice guidelines. *Age Ageing*, 44(1), 25-33.
[http://dx.doi.org/10.1093/ageing/afu143]

OECD. (2017). *Health at a Glance 2017: OECD Indicators..* Paris: OECD Publishing.

Peters, R. (2006). Ageing and the brain. *Postgrad. Med. J., 82*(964), 84-88.
[http://dx.doi.org/10.1136/pgmj.2005.036665] [PMID: 16461469]

Petroianu, A., Capanema, H.X.D.M., Silva, M.M.Q., Braga, N.T.P. (2010). Atividade física e mental no risco de demência em idosos. *J. Bras. Psiquiatr., 59*(4), 302-307.
[http://dx.doi.org/10.1590/S0047-20852010000400006]

PORDATA. (2016). *Indicadores de envelhecimento em Portugal.* Retrieved 10/03/2017 from: http://www.pordata.pt/Portugal/Indicadores+de+envelhecimento-526

PORDATA. (2017). *População residente segundo os Censos: total e por grandes grupos etários – Portugal.* Retrieved 10/03/2017 from: http://www.pordata.pt/Portugal/Popula

PORDATA. (2011). *Base de dados Portugal contemporâneo: população residente.* Retrieved 02/11/2013 from: http://www.pordata.pt/Europa/Populacao+residente-1951

Rimmer, J. (2003). Alzheimer Disease.*Durstine, JL, Moore, GE (org). ACSM's Exercise Management for Persons with Chronic Diseases and Disabilities.* (2nd ed., pp. 311-319). Champaign, IL: Human Kinetics.

Rolland, Y., Pillard, F., Klapouszczak, A., Reynish, E., Thomas, D., Andrieu, S., Rivière, D., Vellas, B. (2007). Exercise program for nursing home residents with Alzheimer's disease: a 1-year randomized, controlled trial. *J. Am. Geriatr. Soc., 55*(2), 158-165.
[http://dx.doi.org/10.1111/j.1532-5415.2007.01035.x] [PMID: 17302650]

Ropper, A.H., Brown, R.H. (2005). *Adams and Victor's - Principles of Neurology* McGraw-Hill - Medical Publishing Division.

Rosa, M. J. (2012). *O Envelhecimento da Sociedade Portuguesa.* Lisboa: Fundação Francisco Manuel dos Santos.

Santana, I., Farinha, F., Freitas, S., Rodrigues, V., Carvalho, Å. (2015). Epidemiologia da Demência e da Doença de Alzheimer em Portugal: Estimativas da Prevalência e dos Encargos Financeiros com a Medicação. *Acta Med. Port., 28*(2), 182-188.
[http://dx.doi.org/10.20344/amp.6025] [PMID: 26061508]

Santos, W., Rabischoffsky, A., Mesquita, C., Costa, R., & Serra, S. (2013). Exames Subsidiários em Cardiogeriatria. In Freitas, E., Py, L., Cançado, F. , Doll, J., & Gorzoni, M. (Eds). *Tratado de geriatria e gerontologia.* Rio de Janeiro: Guanabara Koogan, 2013. Pp. 556-596.

Sarbadhikari, S.N., Saha, A.K. (2006). Moderate exercise and chronic stress produce counteractive effects on different areas of the brain by acting through various neurotransmitter receptor subtypes: a hypothesis. *Theor. Biol. Med. Model., 3*(1), 33.
[http://dx.doi.org/10.1186/1742-4682-3-33] [PMID: 16995950]

Sheehan, B. (2012). Assessment scales in dementia. *Ther. Adv. Neurol. Disorder., 5*(6), 349-358.
[http://dx.doi.org/10.1177/1756285612455733] [PMID: 23139705]

Shimoda, M., Dubas, J., Lira, C. (2007). *Exercício e doença de Alzheimer.* Brasil: Centro de Estudos de Fisiologia do Exercicio.. Available at: http://www.gruponitro.com.br/atendimento-a-profissionais/%23/pdfs/artigos/multidisciplinares/alzheimer.pdf

Sink, K.M., Espeland, M.A., Castro, C.M., Church, T., Cohen, R., Dodson, J.A., Guralnik, J., Hendrie, H.C., Jennings, J., Katula, J., Lopez, O.L., McDermott, M.M., Pahor, M., Reid, K.F., Rushing, J., Verghese, J., Rapp, S., Williamson, J.D. LIFE Study Investigators. (2015). Effect of a 24-month physical activity intervention vs health education on cognitive outcomes in sedentary older adults: the LIFE randomized trial. *JAMA, 314*(8), 781-790.
[http://dx.doi.org/10.1001/jama.2015.9617] [PMID: 26305648]

Stathokostas, L., Little, R.M., Vandervoort, A.A., Paterson, D.H. (2012). Flexibility training and functional ability in older adults: a systematic review. *J. Aging Res., 2012*306818
[http://dx.doi.org/10.1155/2012/306818] [PMID: 23209904]

Suo, C., Singh, M.F., Gates, N., Wen, W., Sachdev, P., Brodaty, H., Saigal, N., Wilson, G.C., Meiklejohn, J., Singh, N., Baune, B.T., Baker, M., Foroughi, N., Wang, Y., Mavros, Y., Lampit, A., Leung, I., Valenzuela, M.J. (2016). Therapeutically relevant structural and functional mechanisms triggered by physical and cognitive exercise. *Mol. Psychiatry, 21*(11), 1633-1642.
[http://dx.doi.org/10.1038/mp.2016.19] [PMID: 27001615]

Sutoo, D., Akiyama, K. (2003). Regulation of brain function by exercise. *Neurobiol. Dis., 13*(1), 1-14.
[http://dx.doi.org/10.1016/S0969-9961(03)00030-5] [PMID: 12758062]

Tabert, M.H., Albert, S.M., Borukhova-Milov, B.A., Camacho, M.S., Pelton, G., Liu, X., Devanand, D.P. (2002). Functional deficits in patients with mild cognitive impairment: prediction of AD. *Neurology, 58*(5), 758-764.

Toots, A., Littbrand, H., Lindelöf, N., Wiklund, R., Holmberg, H., Nordström, P., Lundin-Olsson, L., Gustafson, Y., Rosendahl, E. (2016). Effects of a High-Intensity Functional Exercise Program on Dependence in Activities of Daily Living and Balance in Older Adults with Dementia. *J. Am. Geriatr. Soc., 64*(1), 55-64.
[http://dx.doi.org/10.1111/jgs.13880] [PMID: 26782852]

United Nations - Department of Economic and Social Affairs, Population Division *World Population Ageing 2017 – Highlights..* New York: United Nations. (ST/ESA/SER.A/397).. Available at: https://www.un.org/en/development/desa/population/publications/pdf/ageing/WPA2017_Highlights.pdf

van Praag, H. (2009). Exercise and the brain: something to chew on. *Trends Neurosci., 32*(5), 283-290.

[http://dx.doi.org/10.1016/j.tins.2008.12.007] [PMID: 19349082]

Volchegorskii, I.A., Shemyakov, S.E., Turygin, V.V., Malinovskaya, N.V. (2004). The age dynamics of monoamine oxidase activity and levels of lipid peroxidation products in the human brain. *Neurosci. Behav. Physiol., 34*(4), 303-305.
[http://dx.doi.org/10.1023/B:NEAB.0000018736.84877.4f] [PMID: 15341202]

Vreugdenhil, A., Cannell, J., Davies, A., Razay, G. (2012). A community-based exercise programme to improve functional ability in people with Alzheimer's disease: a randomized controlled trial. *Scand. J. Caring Sci., 26*(1), 12-19.
[http://dx.doi.org/10.1111/j.1471-6712.2011.00895.x] [PMID: 21564154]

Vercambre, M.N., Grodstein, F., Manson, J.E., Stampfer, M.J., Kang, J.H. (2011). Physical activity and cognition in women with vascular conditions. *Arch. Intern. Med., 171*(14), 1244-1250.
[http://dx.doi.org/10.1001/archinternmed.2011.282] [PMID: 21771894]

Wang, L., Larson, E.B., Bowen, J.D., van Belle, G. (2006). Performance-based physical function and future dementia in older people. *Arch. Intern. Med., 166*(10), 1115-1120.
[http://dx.doi.org/10.1001/archinte.166.10.1115] [PMID: 16717174]

Winter, B., Breitenstein, C., Mooren, F.C., Voelker, K., Fobker, M., Lechtermann, A., Krueger, K., Fromme, A., Korsukewitz, C., Floel, A., Knecht, S. (2007). High impact running improves learning. *Neurobiol. Learn. Mem., 87*(4), 597-609.
[http://dx.doi.org/10.1016/j.nlm.2006.11.003] [PMID: 17185007]

World Health Organization. (2015). *Global Action Plan on the Public Health Response to Dementia 2017 - 2025.* Geneva: WHO.

CHAPTER 2

Disorders of Consciousness

Liliana Teixeira[1,*], **Danielle Blacker**[2] and **Nuno Rocha**[3]

[1] *School of Health Sciences; ciTechCare - Center for Innovative Care and Health Technology, CIR - Centre for Rehabilitation Research, Polytechnic of Leiria & Faculdade de Medicina da Universidade de Porto, Portugal*

[2] *Royal Hospital for Neuro-disability, London, UK*

[3] *School of Health, Polytechnic Institute of Porto, Portugal*

Abstract: A disorder of consciousness (DoC) is a state where consciousness has been affected by damage to the brain. DoC range in the form of a hierarchy, including coma, vegetative state and minimally conscious state. The most common way to assess consciousness is to observe their responses to stimulation. However, observing these responses and detecting purposeful behaviours is extremely challenging. Several studies have shown that misdiagnosis is common. It is crucial to optimise the way consciousness assessments are performed. Clinical management of DoC patients, from treatment of pain to end-of-life decisions, depends on behavioural observations. In the present chapter, we review the challenges posed by the assessment of consciousness and the importance of combining clinical assessment with complementary methods of assessment, such as positron emission tomography, functional magnetic resonance imaging and electroencephalography. According to the diagnosis established, the patient will follow different care pathways. Although therapeutic options of DoC are still limited, basic therapies include artificial nutrition and hydration, physical and occupational therapies as well as sensory stimulation. Pharmacologic trials, deep brain stimulation and multisensory stimulations are some of the therapeutic options for DoCs. Recently, it was removed the requirement to obtain legal sanction for every decision to withdraw clinically assisted nutrition and hydration from people in DoCs. This has led to an entire paradigm shift, from a focus on the diagnosis to a focus on the patient's best interest. Although these decisions will spare the courts' involvement, one should never disregard reaching a correct diagnosis for this vulnerable population.

Keywords: Anoxia, Assessment, Brain injury, Coma, Consciousness, Diagnosis, Disorders of consciousness, Emergence, Minimally conscious state, Misdiagnosis, Prognosis, Treatment, Vegetative state.

* **Corresponding author Liliana Teixeira:** School of Health Sciences & ciTechCare - Center for Innovative Care and Health Technology, Polytechnic of Leiria, Portugal; Tel: 00351911549838; E-mail: liliana.teixeira@ipleiria.pt

INTRODUCTION

A brain injury can be classified as traumatic (*i.e.* a car accident or a fall); nontraumatic (*i.e.* drowning, drug overdose, heart attack); and spontaneous (*i.e.* a bleed or virus). The most severe type of acquired brain injury can be classified under the term 'disorders of consciousness' (DoC). DoC can be used to describe a spectrum of disorders, in which consciousness is altered in a transient or permanent way (Monti, 2015). DoC range in the form of a hierarchy, including coma, vegetative state (VS) or a minimally conscious state (MCS).

A DoC, or impaired consciousness, is a state where consciousness has been affected by damage to the brain. Consciousness has two fundamental elements: arousal and awareness. Arousal refers to the level of alertness, determined by eye opening and basic reflexes such as coughing. Awareness is associated with more complex thought processes and the content of consciousness, which is determined by the ability to follow commands or purposeful motor behaviours such as localising and eye-tracking (Laureys *et al.*, 2000).

After extensive brain damage, the surviving patients may only regain limited levels of consciousness. The most common way to assess consciousness is to observe their responses to stimulation. However, observing these responses and detecting purposeful behaviours is extremely challenging. The extensive range of impairments (verbal, motor and cognitive), low arousal levels, medication and lack of assessor experience, contribute to the difficulty in reaching a correct diagnosis (Heine, Laureys, & Schnakers, 2016; Gill-Thwaites, 2006).

DEFINITIONS

Coma

People in a coma are completely unresponsive. They do not move, and their eyes remain closed. The person does not react to external stimuli such as light, sound or pain. It is almost as though the person is under a general anaesthetic. Some patients with very severe brain injuries who do not enter a coma naturally are placed in a medically-induced coma to allow the brain time to heal. A coma usually lasts for less than 2 to 4 weeks, during which time a person may 'wake up' and regain consciousness, or progress into a VS or MCS.

Vegetative State (VS)

The term VS was first coined by Jennett and Plum in 1972. They described it as a paradoxical state of wakefulness without awareness, in which a person has no awareness of themselves, others or their environment. The main difference between 'coma' and VS is that the person in VS has a sleep/wake cycle. They are able to open their eyes and there will be times when they appear to be 'awake'. A person in VS is unable to show meaningful responses to any stimuli. They may move, but this movement is reflexive or spontaneous (non-purposeful). Movements can include grinding their teeth and facial movements such as grimacing. They might jerk as a reflex response to loud noises or move away from a source of pain. They may produce sounds such as grunting. There will be no reproducible, purposeful, or voluntary behavioural responses to visual, auditory, tactile or noxious stimuli and no evidence of language comprehension or expression (Bernat, 2009).

Minimally Conscious State (MCS)

The term MCS was first introduced in 2002, by Giacino *et al.*, (2002) and unlike the VS, MCS is a state of consciousness. This designation enriched the clinical scene, by giving a name to a cohort of patients, who were previously grouped within the VS and whose diagnosis remains confused with it (Fins & Bernat, 2018). A person who is 'minimally conscious' shows some evidence of awareness of themselves or their environment. An example might be the ability to follow simple commands, even if inconsistently. Giacino *et al.*, (2002) quantified MCS as limited and inconsistent but clear evidence of awareness. Some people with brain damage are blind, or deaf, or unable to move certain parts of their bodies, therefore, what a minimally conscious person can do to demonstrate that they are aware of themselves and their environment will vary. There will be times when they can follow simple commands and times when they cannot – their consciousness is likely to fluctuate.

MCS was later subcategorised by Bruno, Vanhaudenhuyse, and Thibaut (2011), based on the complexity of the patients' behaviours. The term MCS+ was used to describe patients with high-level behavioural responses (*i.e.*, patients who can follow commands, have intelligible verbalisations or non-functional communication) and MCS- to describe patients with low-level behavioural responses (*i.e.*, patients who can visual pursuit, localise noxious stimulation or contingent behaviours such as appropriate smiling or crying to emotional stimuli).

Emergence from MCS

Although both VS and MCS are often transitional states between coma and higher levels of consciousness, some patients may fail to fully recover awareness and remain in DoC for the rest of their lives (Estraneo & Trojano, 2018). The Royal College of Physicians (RCP) guidelines for prolonged disorders of consciousness propose that emergence from MCS can be assessed and measured through demonstration of functional communication and functional object use (RCP,

2013). The guidelines suggest the individual should give 6/6 correct yes/no responses on two consecutive occasions. It should be noted that accuracy can be affected by potential language and cognitive impairments. It is therefore important that an experienced and specialised multidisciplinary team of professionals are involved (Pundole & Crawford, 2017). The simplest and most relevant questions should be used (for example object recognition or autobiographical information). Consideration should be given to timely but inaccurate responses, which indicate some awareness that a question is being asked and a response is expected. In terms of functional object use, the RCP guidelines suggest that the individual should use at least two different objects on two consecutive occasions. Difficulties can arise due to lack of motor control, language deficits, sensory impairments. It is recommended that objects offered are familiar everyday objects to facilitate patients to demonstrate their level of awareness by interacting with an object. An occupational therapist is skilled to assess the interactions a person has with an object including how it is held, manipulated and the orientation of the object in relation to the environment.

DIAGNOSIS AND CLINICAL ASSESSMENT

Establishing a proper diagnosis is challenging but of high clinical relevance, as the outcome of a conscious and an unconscious patient is different. The diagnosis also has an impact on also impacts on the care and therapeutic choices, not only regarding pharmacological or non-pharmacological interventions but also regarding therapy. With regards to end-of-life decisions, until very recently, the decision was based on the diagnosis; patients in VS had the legal right to have their artificial nutrition and hydration withdrawn. However, there has been a change in this paradigm. Whereas before, the end-of-life decisions were made based on the diagnosis, now, it is based on the patients' best interests. Nonetheless, a correct diagnosis is always crucial.

Differentiating VS from MCS is challenging since purposeful, spontaneous and reflexive behaviours can be difficult to differentiate and subtle signs of consciousness may be missed. A person in VS might grasp someone's hand reflexively, but a person who is minimally conscious, could perhaps reach for the hand. Unlike most medical conditions, these two are not fixed diagnoses but rather brain states that can evolve. Moreover, the fact that behaviours, which might indicate consciousness in the MCS patient, are manifested episodically and intermittently, it makes the diagnosis of this condition more challenging; and more likely to be missed (Fins, 2016).

Misdiagnosis

Several studies have shown that misdiagnosis of the VS and MCS patients is common. Childs and Mercer (1996) reviewed 193 patients and found that 37% of patients admitted to a rehabilitation unit with a diagnosis of VS were indeed in MCS. The authors have also identified that the misdiagnosis is often due to the lack of extended observation of cognitive awareness by staff with both knowledge and experience in the diagnostic process. A study by Andrews, Murphy, Munday and Littlewood (1996) reported that of the 40 patients admitted with a diagnosis of VS for longer than six months, 43% of the patients had been misdiagnosed, including several patients who were thought to be in VS for several years.

The development of diagnostic criteria for MCS by Giacino *et al.*, (2002) would be expected to reduce the incidence of misdiagnosis relative to the rates reported before these criteria were established. However, recent studies found that still around 40% of patients believed to be in VS were still misdiagnosed. Gill-Thwaites and Munday (2004) found that 45% of the 60 participants in their study were misdiagnosed and Schnakers *et al.*, (2009) identified that 41% of the patients were in MCS rather than VS and out of those that were diagnosed with MCS, 10% had in fact emerged.

Misdiagnosis can and should be avoided; however, it is not always possible or within the assessor's control. Nonetheless, it is particularly crucial to optimise the way consciousness assessments are performed as clinical management of DoC patients, from treatment of pain to end-of-life decisions, depends on behavioural observations. Therefore, the use of standardised and sensitive behavioural assessment scales can noticeably help clinicians to identify subtle signs of consciousness (Heine, Laureys, & Schnakers, 2013).

Behavioural Assessment Scales

A systematic review of behavioural assessment scales of DoCs, conducted by Seel *et al.*, (2009), concluded that Coma Recovery Scale-revised (CRS-r) may be used to assess DoC with minor reservations, and the Sensory Modality Assessment and Rehabilitation Technique (SMART), Wessex Head Injury Matrix (WHIM), and three other less commonly used tools such as the Western Neuro Sensory Stimulation Profile (WNSSP), Sensory Stimulation Assessment Measure (SSAM) and Disorders of Consciousness Scale (DoCS) may be used to assess DoC with moderate reservations. More recently, a study by Godbolt *et al.*, (2010) identified that the CRS-r and SMART established the same level of functioning in 6/10 patients. For the remaining 4, SMART facilitated a higher level of response resulting in the diagnosis of MCS for 3 of the participants and emerging MCS for the fourth. The authors concluded that it is likely that the longer assessment period of SMART, which enabled clinicians to explore consciousness and the use of stimuli pertinent to the patient, may have accounted for this difference.

Clinical assessment is complex and should gather information over time from a variety of sources. It should involve a range of trained and experienced professionals and a selection of different measures. Key observations should include observations from people who know the patient well including caretakers, family and friends. They are potentially more familiar with the patient and their responses. This type of feedback needs careful consideration as observations can be easily misinterpreted such as reflexive eye-watering being interpreted as crying and an emotional response. Diagnosis cannot be based on a single assessment. It is important that observations are repeated and reviewed over an adequate period using a combination of both detailed clinical evaluation and validated, structured assessment tools (RCP, 2013). Diagnosis relies on specialised sensory assessments designed to elicit meaningful responses. It is important that clinical assessment is repeated to ensure that potential awareness is identified and interpreted accurately (Owen and Coleman, 2008).

Neuroimaging

While the assessment scales involve detailed behavioural assessments, they are nevertheless ultimately scored based on the clinicians' subjective opinion of the patients' response (Cruse, Monti, & Owen, 2011). Recent advances in neuroimaging technology may provide a solution for reliance upon behavioural responses when assessing patients with DoC.

Over the past two decades, neuroimaging techniques have contributed enormously in shaping our understanding of DoC. Positron emission tomography (PET), functional magnetic resonance imaging (fMRI) and electroencephalography (EEG) are some of the techniques used to identify consciousness in an unconscious mind (Monti, 2013). These techniques have demonstrated the possibility of cognitive-motor dissociation, detected by fMRI, in which patients who appear behaviourally to be vegetative demonstrate activity on passive and active paradigms with functional studies (Owen *et al.*, 2006). In one case, fMRI was used as a means of functional communication (Monti, Vanhaudenhuyse, & Coleman, 2010). In these papers, the authors were able to produce consistent neural responses to command on behaviourally unresponsive patients. This demonstrates that the clinical diagnoses based on behavioural assessment were inaccurate as they did not accurately reflect the patients' internal states of awareness. Yet, no behavioural marker of awareness was missed by the clinicians. While this neural behaviour does not alter the patient's diagnoses, it demonstrates a level of responsivity that could not be revealed by behavioural scales alone (Cruse, Monti, & Owen, 2011). This complementary assessment method brought major contributions to our knowledge of DoC.

PROGNOSIS

As DoC can result from numerous initial diagnoses, there are currently no reliable statistics on prevalence. Research continues into clinical tools such as fMRI to improve diagnostic accuracy which has prognostic applications.

Three main factors are known to influence the prognosis of patients in VS and MCS: time spent in DoC, age at the time of injury and the nature of the injury (RCP, 2013; Multi-Society Task Force, 1994; Giacino and Kalmar 2005).

- **Time** - The longer a person remains in the state, the less likely recovery of functional improvement becomes (likely related to the severity of brain damage).
- **Age** - Younger patients have a better recovery rate (likely influencing the physiological process of recovery *e.g.* brain plasticity).
- **Type** - The cause of injury plays a significant prognostic role. A non-traumatic (anoxic or diffuse) injury has a shorter window for potential recovery and is associated with greater severity of disability than patients with a traumatic aetiology.
- The presence of clinical complications that could impact care strategies will also influence the likelihood of functional improvement.

Based on a large cohort analysis, the MSTF (1994), reported on the probability of recovering full consciousness following DoC, as being very low beyond 12 months after traumatic brain injury (TBI) and 3 months after non-traumatic injury. The RCP guidelines (2013) recommended a more cautious period of 6 months for non-traumatic brain injury. Based on these considerations, the term "permanent" VS was proposed, to classify VS patients in apparently irreversible unconscious clinical state. At that time, only occasional case reports were available about the late recovery of consciousness beyond the above temporal limits. However, likely due to improvements in preventive and restorative therapeutic strategies, ideas on clinical evolution in DoC patients progressively changed. In 1995, the American Congress of Rehabilitation Medicine suggested avoiding time-based prognostic statements *i.e.* not to use the term "permanent." Since then, case reports and cohort studies have documented the late recovery of variable levels of consciousness beyond the timeframes specified even in vascular and anoxic VS patients. It is therefore, important to view the temporal definitions as probabilities to identify the point after which recovery of consciousness is 'highly improbable' but not impossible. A guideline update, published in 2018, suggests that the term chronic should replace permanent VS (Giacino *et al.*, 2018). For those patients who regain some level of consciousness later, improvements are often minimal, and most patients are affected by severe functional disability. These findings would suggest that some kind of brain plasticity could not be excluded even for a long time after a severe brain injury. However, the occurrence of severe motor and cognitive deficits suggests there is a need for early appropriate levels of rehabilitation. This could facilitate recovery of responsiveness and minimise disabilities (*e.g.* contractures) that negatively influence functional independence and quality of life (Estraneo & Trojano, 2018).

The prognosis for recovery is better for MCS than for VS (Luaute *et al.*, 2010). The MSTF (1994) acknowledges that perhaps 20% of vegetative patients will evolve into MCS. For patients in VS, the large majority of those who regain consciousness have done so by 12 months for traumatic brain injury, and by 3 months for non-traumatic injury (Hirschberg & Giacino, 2011). Most reported cases of patients who have emerged from MCS have done so by 2 years after injury, with the rest regaining consciousness at 2–4 years (Hirschberg & Giacino, 2011). There are isolated reports of recovery of consistent consciousness even after many years, but these are a rarity. Inevitably, those who do "recover" remain profoundly disabled. Any progression is likely to be gradual, and it is likely that patients emerging late from VS/MCS may have shown signs of increasing responsiveness over time.

Clinical predictions about outcome are challenging. Some preliminary studies were conducted with the hopes of using behavioural observations to detect the potential for later emergence from VS (da Conceição Teixeira, Gill-Thwaites, & Reynolds, 2016). The results suggest that the patients who emerged from VS, exhibited a significantly higher number of different behaviours at rest, than those who remained in VS. However, conclusive information is needed to guide clinicians and families in decision-making or to identify patients with potential for recovery (Estraneo & Trojano, 2018). Experts agree that re-evaluation should occur at regular intervals (6 and 12 months, and yearly thereafter) to detect any changes in patients' responsiveness, and such evaluation needs to occur when the patient is physically well. Following the publication of the RCP guidelines (2013), patients diagnosed with VS or MCS are more likely to get such re-evaluations. There are unknown number of patients in nursing homes or the community who have not been formally re-evaluated since their initial diagnosis. Without re-evaluation, the transition from VS to MCS may go unnoticed. Regularly updating diagnoses is critical to determine prognosis, direct appropriate rehabilitation and decisions about withdrawal of treatment (RCP, 2013).

TREATMENT

The RCP guidelines (2013) suggest that a national registry of long-term follow-up data is needed in order to create an evidence base to better understand the benefit of treatment interventions. There are numerous medical and surgical interventions initially available for the treatment of a brain injury. Once a DoC has been established, these guidelines recommend that patients should be admitted to specialist rehabilitation centres for assessment and treatment. The focus being upon maximising a person's potential to demonstrate awareness and preventing secondary complications such as infections or muscle shortening (contractures). To prevent or limit complications, 24-hour care involving a range of specialities is required. Expertise can include: artificial nutritional support, chest physiotherapy, management of surgical airways (tracheostomies), physio- and occupational therapy to manage tone and contractures and the provision of specialised equipment such as seating supports. Sitting in a wheelchair helps increase a patients' levels of arousal and potential to interact (Wilson, Dhamapurkar, & Tunnard, 2014). Specialist care also includes assessments of whether patients can communicate and interact and whether they may be suffering from pain or depression, about which they cannot communicate. Many believed if there was no potential for recovery then there was no logical reason why rehabilitation should take place (Andrews, 1993). However, there is some evidence that early and increased intervention leads to better outcomes (Shiel *et al.*, 2001). Many studies have shown that patients in VS can demonstrate varying degrees of recovery several years post-injury (Elliot & Walker, 2005). The literature on the treatment of DoC patients is divided broadly into two categories: pharmacological and non-pharmacological interventions.

Pharmacological Interventions - Several pharmacological trials have demonstrated benefits of using neuro-stimulant drugs such as Amantadine (a dopaminergic agent) to accelerate the pace of functional recovery and to increase a patient's responsiveness. Several therapeutic trials have been conducted using Zolpidem with post-comatose patients (Machado, Estévez, & Rodriguez-Rojas, 2018). Zolpidem is a drug originally used in the treatment of insomnia that occasionally has an opposite effect in brain-damaged patients. The results varied from a marked improvement in the level of arousal to an enhancement of motor, verbal and cognitive functions (Noormandi, Shahrokhi, & Khalili, 2017). Other pharmacological agents that have been reported as inducing functional recovery are Levodopa, Bromocriptine (Passler & Riggs, 2001), Apomorphine (Fridman *et al.*, 2010) and Baclofen (Taira & Hori, 2007). Large scale studies on the efficacy of these drugs are still warranted.

Non-pharmacological Interventions - Evidence from studies has illustrated that sensory deprivation leads to physical deterioration (Grossman & Hagel, 1996). Many brain-injured patients with sensorimotor impairments have associated motor-related disabilities (Dobkin, 2003). Environmental stimulation routines generally employ sensory stimulation (*e.g.* massage or listening to music) with the aim of increasing the level of arousal and responsiveness to enhance the potential for interaction with one's environment *i.e.* using assistive technologies to request attention (Di Stefano *et al.*, 2012). Sensory regulation is a variant of sensory stimulation that facilitates information processing (Wood *et al.*, 1992). Stimulation sessions are alternated with rest periods in order to increase the ability to respond. More recently, brain stimulation strategies have been used with DoC patients. Deep brain stimulation (DBS) is a surgical procedure where electrodes are implanted in the brain to reactivate cerebral connectivity. Extradural cortical stimulation uses a similar concept where a stimulation lead is placed under local anaesthesia in the epidural space. Similarly, transcranial magnetic stimulation (TMS) is a non-invasive procedure utilising electro-magnetic fields *via* the scalp for neurostimulation. All have been associated with improvements in arousal, motor and verbal functions in some patients (Schiff *et al.* 2007; Laureys *et al.*, 2000; Thibaut & Laureys, 2015). However, the beneficial effects of all these techniques are still debated and are not yet based on evidence or quantifiable improvement of long-term outcomes. Research into treatment is difficult. No animal model exists where meaningful changes in consciousness can be assessed, and DoC patients by definition cannot consent to a trial: interventions that are invasive or where the risks are unknown give rise to significant ethical concerns.

ETHICAL ISSUES

Patients with DoCs are vulnerable to misdiagnosis and to medical mismanagement that can negatively affect their access to ongoing care, rehabilitation and pain medication (Gosseries *et al.*, 2011). Therefore, the management of this population inevitably raises important ethical and legal considerations.

In many countries, it is legally permitted to withdraw artificial nutrition and hydration once the patient is diagnosed as being in a permanent VS, and therefore with no hope of recovery, if it is proved that the withdrawal seems likely to be what the patient would have wanted (Jennet, 2005). Withdrawal of artificial nutrition and hydration from a patient in a VS was given court approval for the first time (in England) in 1993 (Kitzinger & Kitzinger, 2013).

Treatment decisions should be guided by reliable information about how the patient would wish to be treated in this condition (Lochlainn, Gubbins, & Connolly, 2013). Clinicians can obtain this information in advance directives if they exist, and through consultation with the relatives, legal guardian and general practitioner.

Last year, it was removed the requirement to obtain legal sanction for every decision to withdraw clinically assisted nutrition and hydration from people in

DoCs. This has led to an entire paradigm shift, from a focus on the diagnosis to a focus on the patient's best interest (Wade, 2018). The decision making was taken away from the supreme courts to the hands of the clinicians and families. It is believed that the existing law and guidance are enough to ensure good practice. And effective procedures should be adopted to take care of the comatose patient (Wade, 2018). Clinical teams must always include families in decision making from the very beginning. The central feature of this new process is that the team must always establish what the patient would have wanted.

CONCLUSION

Signs of consciousness may be variable and fluctuating. Any recovery can be slow and uncertain and therefore, any signs of awareness may be hard to interpret. It is important for clinicians and assessors to consider that a person's abilities may also be limited by motor or sensory disabilities and impairments. Responses can be delayed or inconsistent due to medical instability, fatigue, communication or cognitive impairments. Before concluding that a patient is vegetative and not minimally conscious, it is important to rule out the possibility that their consciousness is being suppressed by sedative medication or illness. Individuals should be regularly monitored and reviewed to ensure needs are being met and any changes in presentation and ability are identified. One should not forget that neuroimaging technology can provide a measure of the levels of awareness that DoC patients might retain, and most importantly, they overcome the need for these patients to produce discernible behaviours by relying on their mindset as instructed in the paradigm tasks (Cruse, Monti, & Owen, 2011). In the absence of a state of consciousness, the cortical processing that can be detected by neuroimaging techniques is understood to be insufficient to give rise to the subjective feeling of perception. Therefore, the person might be unconscious, but not just vegetative (Monti, 2013).

The rate of misdiagnosis of DoC patients, 4 out of 10, is unthinkable in other medical conditions (Fins & Wright, 2018). Standardised behavioural assessment scales should, therefore, be used routinely by clinicians in order to minimise the risk of misdiagnosis.

Furthermore, DoC patients have limited therapeutic options. Basic therapies include artificial nutrition and hydration, physical and occupational therapies as well as sensory stimulation that are used in the hopes to prevent complications and enhance recovery. Pharmacologic trials have shown behavioral improvements in some uncontrolled case reports or series of brain-injured patients. Deep brain stimulation and multisensory stimulations also showed some positive results but more clinical trials are required (Gosseries *et al.*, 2011).

It is hoped that with the new paradigm shift with regards to the withdrawal of artificial hydration and nutrition, the patients will still have their wishes established and respected. As clinicians, it is of utmost importance to act on the patients' best interests at all times. These decisions will spare the courts' involvement; however, one should never disregard reaching a correct diagnosis and prognosis.

CONSENT FOR PUBLICATION

Not applicable.

CONFLICT OF INTEREST

The author confirms that this chapter contents have no conflict of interest.

ACKNOWLEDGEMENTS

Declared none.

REFERENCES

Andrews, K. (1993). Recovery of patients after four months or more in the persistent vegetative state. *BMJ, 306*(6892), 1597-1600.
[http://dx.doi.org/10.1136/bmj.306.6892.1597] [PMID: 8329926]

Andrews, K., Murphy, L., Munday, R., Littlewood, C. (1996). Misdiagnosis of the vegetative state: retrospective study in a rehabilitation unit. *BMJ, 313*(7048), 13-16.
[http://dx.doi.org/10.1136/bmj.313.7048.13] [PMID: 8664760]

Bernat, J.L. (2009). Chronic consciousness disorders. *Annu. Rev. Med., 60*, 381-392.
[http://dx.doi.org/10.1146/annurev.med.60.060107.091250] [PMID: 19630578]

Bruno, M.A., Vanhaudenhuyse, A., Thibaut, A., Moonen, G., Laureys, S. (2011). From unresponsive wakefulness to minimally conscious PLUS and functional locked-in syndromes: recent advances in our understanding of disorders of consciousness. *J. Neurol., 258*(7), 1373-1384.
[http://dx.doi.org/10.1007/s00415-011-6114-x] [PMID: 21674197]

Childs, N.L., Mercer, W.N. (1996). Misdiagnosing the persistent vegetative state. Misdiagnosis certainly occurs. *BMJ, 313*(7062), 944. [letter, comment].
[http://dx.doi.org/10.1136/bmj.313.7062.944] [PMID: 8876118]

Cruse, D., Monti, M.M., Owen, A. (2011). Neuroimaging in disorders of consciousness: contributions to diagnosis and prognosis. *Future Neurol., 6*(2). https://pdfs.semanticscholar.org/d860/950744f6607 e784d064ed3c0c0cf4a0c2d83.pdf
[http://dx.doi.org/10.2217/fnl.10.87]

da Conceição Teixeira, L., Gill-Thwaites, H., Reynolds, F., Duport, S. (2018). Can behavioural observations made during the SMART assessment detect the potential for later emergence from vegetative state? *Neuropsychol. Rehabil., 28*(8), 1340-1349.
[http://dx.doi.org/10.1080/09602011.2016.1243482] [PMID: 27788632]

Di Stefano, C., Cortesi, A., Masotti, S., Simoncini, L., Piperno, R. (2012). Increased behavioural responsiveness with complex stimulation in VS and MCS: preliminary results. *Brain Inj., 26*(10), 1250-1256.
[http://dx.doi.org/10.3109/02699052.2012.667588] [PMID: 22616735]

Dobkin, B.H. (2003). Do electrically stimulated sensory inputs and movements lead to long-term plasticity and rehabilitation gains? *Curr. Opin. Neurol., 16*(6), 685-691.
[http://dx.doi.org/10.1097/00019052-200312000-00007] [PMID: 14624077]

Elliott, L., Walker, L. (2005). Rehabilitation interventions for vegetative and minimally conscious patients. *Neuropsychol. Rehabil., 15*(3-4), 480-493.
[http://dx.doi.org/10.1080/09602010443000506] [PMID: 16350989]

Estraneo, A. & Trojano, L. (2018). Prognosis in Disorders of Consciousness. In: C. Schnackers & S. Laureys (Eds.), *Coma and Disorders of Consciousness* (pp.17-36).
[http://dx.doi.org/10.1007/978-3-319-55964-3_2]

Fins, J.J., Wright, M.S. (2018). Rights language and disorders of consciousness: a call for advocacy. *Brain Inj., 32*(5), 670-674.
[http://dx.doi.org/10.1080/02699052.2018.1430377] [PMID: 29393694]

Fins, J.J. (2016). Neuroethics and disorders of consciousness: discerning brain states in clinical practice and research. *AMA J. Ethics, 18*(12), 1182-1191.
[http://dx.doi.org/10.1001/journalofethics.2016.18.12.ecas2-1612] [PMID: 28009244]

Fins, J.J., Bernat, J.L. (2018). Ethical, palliative, and policy considerations in disorders of consciousness. *Neurology, 91*(10), 471-475.
[http://dx.doi.org/10.1212/WNL.0000000000005927] [PMID: 30089621]

Fridman, E.A., Krimchansky, B.Z., Bonetto, M., Galperin, T., Gamzu, E.R., Leiguarda, R.C., Zafonte, R. (2010). Continuous subcutaneous apomorphine for severe disorders of consciousness after traumatic brain injury. *Brain Inj., 24*(4), 636-641.
[http://dx.doi.org/10.3109/02699051003610433] [PMID: 20235766]

Giacino, J.T., Kalmar, K. (2005). Diagnostic and prognostic guidelines for the vegetative and minimally conscious states. *Neuropsychol. Rehabil., 15*(3-4), 166-174.
[http://dx.doi.org/10.1080/09602010443000498] [PMID: 16350959]

Giacino, J.T., Ashwal, S., Childs, N., Cranford, R., Jennett, B., Katz, D.I., Kelly, J.P., Rosenberg, J.H., Whyte, J., Zafonte, R.D., Zasler, N.D. (2002). The minimally conscious state: definition and diagnostic criteria. *Neurology, 58*(3), 349-353.
[http://dx.doi.org/10.1212/WNL.58.3.349] [PMID: 11839831]

Giacino, J.T., Katz, D.I., Schiff, N.D., Whyte, J., Armstrong,, M.J. (2018). Practice guideline update recommendations summary: Disorders of consciousness: Report of the Guideline Development, Dissemination, and Implementation Subcommittee of the American Academy of Neurology; the American Congress of Rehabilitation Medicine; and the National Institute on Disability, Independent Living, and Rehabilitation Research. *Neurology, 91*(19), 450-460.
[http://dx.doi.org/10.1212/WNL.0000000000005926.]

Gill-Thwaites, H. (2006). Lotteries, loopholes and luck: misdiagnosis in the vegetative state patient. *Brain Inj., 20*(13-14), 1321-1328.
[http://dx.doi.org/10.1080/02699050601081802] [PMID: 17378223]

Gill-Thwaites, H., Munday, R. (2004). The Sensory Modality Assessment and Rehabilitation Technique (SMART): a valid and reliable assessment for vegetative state and minimally conscious state patients. *Brain Inj., 18*(12), 1255-1269.
[http://dx.doi.org/10.1080/02699050410001719952] [PMID: 15666569]

Godbolt, A.K., Stenson, S., Winberg, M., Tengvar, C. (2012). Disorders of consciousness: preliminary data supports added value of extended behavioural assessment. *Brain Inj., 26*(2), 188-193.
[http://dx.doi.org/10.3109/02699052.2011.648708] [PMID: 22360525]

Gosseries, O., Vanhaudenhuyse, A., Bruno, M.A., Demertzi, A. (2011). Disorders of consciousness: Coma, vegetative and minimally conscious states. In: D. Cvetkovic and I. Cosic (Eds.), *States of Consciousness* (pp.29-55).

[http://dx.doi.org/10.1007/978-3-642-18047-7_2]

Grossman, P., Hagel, K. (1996). Post-traumatic apallic syndrome following head injury. Part 1: clinical characteristics. *Disabil. Rehabil., 18*(1), 1-20.
[http://dx.doi.org/10.3109/09638289609167084] [PMID: 8932740]

Heine, L., Laureys, S., Schnakers, C. (2013). Behavioral Responsiveness in Patients with Disorders of Consciousness. In: Monti, M. M., Sannita, A.G., (Eds.), *Brain Function and Responsiveness in Disorders of Consciousness* (pp. 25-36). Switzerland: Springer International Publishing.
[http://dx.doi.org/10.1007/978-3-319-21425-2_3]

Hirschberg, R., Giacino, J.T. (2011). The vegetative and minimally conscious states: diagnosis, prognosis and treatment. *Neurol. Clin., 29*(4), 773-786.
[http://dx.doi.org/10.1016/j.ncl.2011.07.009] [PMID: 22032660]

Jennett, B., Plum, F. (1972). Persistent vegetative state after brain damage. A syndrome in search of a name. *Lancet, 1*(7753), 734-737.
[http://dx.doi.org/10.1016/S0140-6736(72)90242-5] [PMID: 4111204]

Jennett, B. (2005). 30 Years of the Vegetative State: Clinical, Ethical and Legal Problems.*The Boundaries of Consciousness: Neurobiology and Neuropathology.* (pp. 537-543). Amsterdam: Elsevier.
[http://dx.doi.org/10.1016/S0079-6123(05)50037-2]

Kitzinger, J., Kitzinger, C. (2013). The 'window of opportunity' for death after severe brain injury: family experiences. *Sociol. Health Illn., 35*(7), 1095-1112.
[http://dx.doi.org/10.1111/1467-9566.12020] [PMID: 23278317]

Laureys, S., Faymonville, M.E., Luxen, A., Lamy, M., Franck, G., Maquet, P. (2000). Restoration of thalamocortical connectivity after recovery from persistent vegetative state. *Lancet, 355*(9217), 1790-1791.
[http://dx.doi.org/10.1016/S0140-6736(00)02271-6] [PMID: 10832834]

Luauté, J., Maucort-Boulch, D., Tell, L., Quelard, F., Sarraf, T., Iwaz, J., Boisson, D., Fischer, C. (2010). Long-term outcomes of chronic minimally conscious and vegetative states. *Neurology, 75*(3), 246-252.
[http://dx.doi.org/10.1212/WNL.0b013e3181e8e8df] [PMID: 20554940]

Machado, C., Estévez, M., Rodriguez-Rojas, R. (2018). Zolpidem efficacy and safety in disorders of consciousness. *Brain Inj., 32*(4), 530-531.
[http://dx.doi.org/10.1080/02699052.2018.1429664] [PMID: 29393689]

Monti, M.M., Vanhaudenhuyse, A., Coleman, M.R., Boly, M., Pickard, J.D., Tshibanda, L., Owen, A.M., Laureys, S. (2010). Willful modulation of brain activity in disorders of consciousness. *N. Engl. J. Med., 362*(7), 579-589.
[http://dx.doi.org/10.1056/NEJMoa0905370] [PMID: 20130250]

Monti, M.M. (2013). Editorial – Ethics, neuroimaging and disorders of consciousness: What is the question? *Am. J. Bioeth., 4*(4), 1-2.
[PMID: 23514383]

Monti, M.M. (2015). Disorders of Consciousness. *Emerging Trends in the Social and Behavioral Sciences.* Hoboken, NJ: John Wiley & Sons.
[http://dx.doi.org/10.1002/9781118900772.etrds0077]

Ní Lochlainn, M., Gubbins, S., Connolly, S., Reilly, R.B. (2013). The vegetative and minimally conscious states: a review of the literature and preliminary survey of prevalence in Ireland. *Ir. J. Med. Sci., 182*(1), 7-15. [http://dx.doi.org/10.1007/s11845-012-0825-6] [PMID: 22528253]

Noormandi, A., Shahrokhi, M., Khalili, H. (2017). Potential benefits of zolpidem in disorders of consciousness. *Expert Rev. Clin. Pharmacol., 10*(9), 983-992.
[http://dx.doi.org/10.1080/17512433.2017.1347502] [PMID: 28649875]

Owen, A.M., Coleman, M.R. (2008). Detecting awareness in the vegetative state. *Ann. N. Y. Acad. Sci., 1129*, 130-138.

[http://dx.doi.org/10.1196/annals.1417.018] [PMID: 18591475]

Owen, A.M., Coleman, M.R., Boly, M., Davis, M.H., Laureys, S., Pickard, J.D. (2006). Detecting awareness in the vegetative state. *Science, 313*(5792), 1402.
[http://dx.doi.org/10.1126/science.1130197] [PMID: 16959998]

Passler, M.A., Riggs, R.V. (2001). Positive outcomes in traumatic brain injury-vegetative state: patients treated with bromocriptine. *Arch. Phys. Med. Rehabil., 82*(3), 311-315.
[http://dx.doi.org/10.1053/apmr.2001.20831] [PMID: 11245751]

Pundole, A., Crawford, S. (2018). The assessment of language and the emergence from disorders of consciousness. *Neuropsychol. Rehabil., 28*(8), 1285-1294.
[http://dx.doi.org/10.1080/09602011.2017.1307766] [PMID: 28385064]

Royal College of Physicians. (2013). Prolonged disorders of consciousness: National clinical guidelines. London: Royal College of Physicians Retrieved from: https://www.rcplondon.ac.uk/guidelines-policy/prolonged-disorders-consciousness-national-clinical-guidelines

Schiff, N.D., Giacino, J.T., Kalmar, K., Victor, J.D., Baker, K., Gerber, M., Fritz, B., Eisenberg, B., Biondi, T., O'Connor, J., Kobylarz, E.J., Farris, S., Machado, A., McCagg, C., Plum, F., Fins, J.J., Rezai, A.R. (2007). Behavioural improvements with thalamic stimulation after severe traumatic brain injury. *Nature, 448*(7153), 600-603.
[http://dx.doi.org/10.1038/nature06041] [PMID: 17671503]

Schnakers, C., Vanhaudenhuyse, A., Giacino, J., Ventura, M., Boly, M., Majerus, S., Moonen, G., Laureys, S. (2009). Diagnostic accuracy of the vegetative and minimally conscious state: clinical consensus *versus* standardized neurobehavioral assessment. *BMC Neurol., 9*, 35.
[http://dx.doi.org/10.1186/1471-2377-9-35] [PMID: 19622138]

Seel, R.T., Sherer, M., Whyte, J., Katz, D.I., Giacino, J.T., Rosenbaum, A.M., Hammond, F.M., Kalmar, K., Pape, T.L., Zafonte, R., Biester, R.C., Kaelin, D., Kean, J., Zasler, N. (2010). Assessment scales for disorders of consciousness: evidence-based recommendations for clinical practice and research. *Arch. Phys. Med. Rehabil., 91*(12), 1795-1813.
[http://dx.doi.org/10.1016/j.apmr.2010.07.218] [PMID: 21112421]

Shiel, A., Burn, J.P., Henry, D., Clark, J., Wilson, B.A., Burnett, M.E., McLellan, D.L. (2001). The effects of increased rehabilitation therapy after brain injury: results of a prospective controlled trial. *Clin. Rehabil., 15*(5), 501-514.
[http://dx.doi.org/10.1191/026921501680425225] [PMID: 11594640]

Taira, T., Hori, T. (2007). Diaphragm pacing with a spinal cord stimulator: current state and future directions. *Acta Neurochir. Suppl. (Wien), 97*(Pt 1), 289-292.
[PMID: 17691389]

The Multi-Society Task Force report on PVS (1994). Medical aspects of the persistent vegetative state (1). *New Engl. J. Med., 330*(21), 1499-508.

Thibaut, A., Laureys, S. (2015). Brain stimulation in patients with disorders of consciousness. *Princ. Pract. Clin. Res., 1*(3), 65-75.

Wade, D. (2018). Editorial – Clinically assisted nutrition and hydration. *BMJ, 361*https://www.bmj.com/content/362/bmj.k3869

Wilson, B., Dhamapurkar, S., Tunnard, C., Watson, P. (2014). The effect of positioning on the level of arousal and awareness in patients in the vegetative state or the minimally conscious state: a replication and extension of a previous finding. *Brain Impair., 14*(3), 475-479.
[http://dx.doi.org/10.1017/BrImp.2013.34]

Wood, R.L., Winkowski, T.B., Miller, J.L., Tierney, L., Goldman, L. (1992). Evaluating sensory regulation as a method to improve awareness in patients with altered states of consciousness: a pilot study. *Brain Inj., 6*(5), 411-418.
[http://dx.doi.org/10.3109/02699059209008137] [PMID: 1393174]

CHAPTER 3

Promoting Autonomous Language Learning in People with Special Needs: Universal Design for Learning in the Project En-Abilities

Sergio Sanchez[1]**, José Luis González**[2]**, Elena Alcalde**[3]**, Jaime Ribeiro**[4,5,*]**, Margarida Lucas**[5] **and António Moreira**[5]

[1] *Interfaculty Department of Evolutionary Psychology and Education, Autonomous University of Madrid, Spain*

[2] *University of Burgos, Education Faculty, Spain*

[3] *Departament of Modern Philology, University of Alcalá, Madrid, Spain*

[4] *School of Health Sciences & ciTechCare - Center for Innovative Care and Health Technology, Polytechnic of Leiria, Portugal*

[5] *CIDTFF - Research Centre on Didactics and Technology in the Education of Trainers - University of Aveiro, Portugal*

Abstract: The international society is involved in an active commercial and labour activity. This activity is based on the elimination of barriers and the dissipation of borders. Everyone wants their part of the European dream, but not everyone has equal opportunities and fair access. People with disabilities or other needs often encounter obstacles, including difficulty or inability to communicate in a non-native language, English. This chapter presents the EN-ABILITIES Project that seeks the inclusion of human diversity through communication in English. Here, we present a survey of English learning needs by people with special needs, as well as a structure for an online accessible learning model. A review of European legislation and the different concepts of universal design applied to learning contexts is presented, as well as the results of a placement test conducted with people people with disabilities and the perspectives of English teachers about the teaching of this language to people with disabilities. It also addresses the particularities to be taken into account when providing online training for people with diverse skills.

Keywords: Autonomous language learning, EN-ABILITIES, People with special needs, Universal design for learning.

[*] **Corresponding author Jaime Ribeiro:** Research Centre on Didactics and Technology in the Education of Trainers - University of Aveiro, Portugal; Tel: +34 91 497 3155; E-mail: jaimeribeiro@ua.pt

Samuel Honório, Marco Batista, Helena Mesquita & Jaime Ribeiro (Eds.)

INTRODUCTION

More often than what should be desired in our society, buildings, software or information systems - to name just a few - are usually developed for prototypical users, leading to the neglect of users with disabilities and/or Special Educational Needs (SEN) (Sanchez, Diez & Martin, 2015). Fortunately, throughout the twentieth century, changes that have taken place in society have led to the adoption of new paradigms that have improved the situation of people with disabilities (Preiser & Ostroff, 2001). It is in this context that what is known as the paradigm of Universal Design was born, although it was not until the beginning of the new century, specifically in 2001, when its first handbook was published (Preiser & Ostroff, 2001). The publication of this reference showed that, in the realm of design, a significant number of changes had taken place and that it was necessary to have documents and resources which could act as guidelines for professionals in this field. Since then, the technological, economic, social, and even legal spheres have modified the discourse of the practice of universal design in society (Preiser & Smith, 2011). In addition, the rights of people with disabilities have been acknowledged by most people and governments over the last decade in relation to what accessibility and universal design refers to. Therefore, the need and obligation of teaching that complies with the social mandates to address diversity is becoming increasingly necessary.

Since its formulation, universal design and other similar concepts have described the complexity, dynamism and reciprocity of the relationship between the environment and the person (Webb & Hoover, 2015). In addition, universal design has become significant in the formation of legislation. The European base in terms of accessibility – pre-dating the concept of universal design - took place in 1988 with the launch of the HELIOS program. As a continuation of this first program, in the year 1996, subsequent studies within HELIOS II were complemented. The objectives of both projects were to promote the social and economic integration of people with disabilities, as well as to promote the possibility of achieving the basis for living an independent life (Zolkowska, Kasior-Szerszen & Blaszkiewicz, 2002).

More recently, the field of universal design has acquired a wide presence in Spanish legislation. The laws enacted throughout the last decade have greatly favoured the promotion and dissemination of the philosophy derived from these concepts. The fundamental law by which people with disabilities are guaranteed their rights in the Spanish state already refers to the need for accessibility and design for everyone in its own title. While it is true that, at present, the law that encompasses these rights is the General Law on the Rights of Persons with Disabilities and their Social Inclusion, it is the previous legislation that includes all the normative development of this idea. Therefore, it was Law 51/2003, of December 2nd, 2003, on equal opportunities, non-discrimination and universal accessibility for people with disabilities which changed the view which society and its members had on how to address diversity.

Throughout this legal text-specific references are made to accessibility and design for all as basic tools. Thus, in Article 2, Principles, the concepts of universal accessibility and design for all are well detailed. These terms will be constantly used later throughout the norm. These definitions are as follows:

"c) universal accessibility: the condition that environments, processes, goods, products and services must meet, as well as objects or instruments, tools and devices, to be understandable, usable and practicable by all people in conditions of safety and comfort and in the most autonomous and natural way possible. It presupposes the strategy of "design for all" and is understood without prejudice to the reasonable adjustments that must be adopted.

d) design for all: the activity by which it is conceived or projected, from its inception, and whenever possible, environments, processes, goods, products, services, objects, instruments, devices or tools, in such a way that they can be used by all people, to the greatest extent possible. "

Both terms constitute the basis of all the normative principles used later in the rest of Spanish legislation. These are the same terms used in the international declaration of the rights of persons with disabilities, in the objectives of sustainable development and the 2030 agenda, as well as in the European 2010-2020 and Spanish 2012-2020 disability strategies.

Regarding the educational context, the concept and idea of the design for all is also clearly validated. The Organic Law 8/2013, of December 9, 2013, for the improvement of the quality of education in Spain describes the need to serve everyone with a model based on inclusion and with principles of universality, design for all and accessibility. The Organic Law 4/2007, of April 12, 2007, which modifies the Organic Law 6/2001, of December 21, 2001, referring to tertiary or university level studies, mentions in its twenty-fourth additional provision that there is an obligation to consider universal design criteria in higher education. In addition, and to conclude this review of the legislative context related to universal design, we must highlight the provisions of the Royal Decree 1393/2007, of October 29, 2007, which established the organization of the official university education in Spain. In its preamble, this law states that training in any professional activity should contribute to the knowledge and development of Human Rights, democratic principles, the principles of equality between women and men, solidarity, enviornmental protection, universal accessibility and design for all, and the promotion of a culture of peace.

As we can see, Spanish legislation stresses the importance of fostering the inclusion of learners with Special Educational Needs within the formal educational settings and as a direct consequence of supporting a greater inclusion of these participants within everyday life and activities of Spanish society. Nevertheless, a question that arises is under which concepts and theoretical basis is this inclusion supported. To answer this question, we will now refer to the idea of universal design as the means of creating content which is appropriate for all members of a given society.

UNIVERSAL DESIGN: DEFINITION AND MAIN CONCEPTS

As we have already seen, an important aspect of the quest for universal inclusion and accessibility of learners within the educational system and context, both formal, non-formal or informal, is the idea surrounding the concept of universal design. As indicated by Story (2011), the appearance of varied terminology around universal design is a sign of the good health of the concept and the work that is carried out within this scientific area. Regardless of the specific denomination, the final common goal of different denominated streams with different verbal labels is to achieve accessibility for as many people as possible from the initial moments of design and construction of any idea, project or concept. Historically, the use of the different terms has been linked to the geographical area in which each of them has been applied (Sanchez, *et al.*, 2015), and the cultural differences are evident in the terminology that has been developed (Ostroff, 2011, cited in Webb, Williams & Smith, 2011). While different theories have sought to envisage the different links between social and physical factors in explaining the concept (*e.g.*, Altman and Chemer, 1984, Bronfenbrenner, 2005, Gibson, 1977, Lawton & Nahemow, 2010, cited in Webb, *et al.*, 2011), three primary ideas have gained most traction:

"In the first place, no single theory considers all the complexity of the relationship between person-environment; secondly, the person-environment construct is constantly changing in relation to the personal circumstances of each person (*e.g.*, age, environmental factors, mobility, *etc.*), therefore, it is a dynamic and not stagnant concept; and thirdly, technical, economic, social and environmental changes have led to innovation in design and ideological changes in society." (Webb, *et al.*, 2011, p.440).

Those concepts that have had a greater significance in different areas, and that have been studied and developed by research teams in the main international research centres, are considered of special importance. In this sense, some denominations, such as accessible design (Iwarsson & Stahl, 2003) or usable design (ISO, 1998), can be included within higher categories.

If the above-mentioned ideas are transferred to the educational field, we also witness that the concept of universal design has been transformed and studied from different perspectives. As Sala, Sánchez, Gine & Diez (2014) stated, during the process of creating this new educational paradigm, different application approaches with different and similar names have emerged, especially within the Anglo-Saxon context. The four main paradigms in the application of universal design to educational spaces are: (a) Universal Design for Learning; (b) Universal Instructional Design; (c) Universal Design for Instruction; and (d) Universal Design in Education.

In Table **1**, we include Sala *et al.*'s (2014) summary of the four main paradigms, their principles, development centres and main authors.

Nevertheless, these theoretical ideas of universal design must be applied to specific contexts and situations if they are to be useful in the quest for global inclusion of participants in situations of vulnerability. In the next section, we will present a specific trans-European project in which the aim is to support people with Special Educational Needs acquire enough proficiency in a second language to increase their possibilities of social inclusion and obtaining a job.

EN-ABILITIES PROJECT: SUPPORTING LEARNERS WITH SEN ACQUIRE A SECOND LANGUAGE

Currently, educational instruction is not restricted to classroom courses which require face to face interaction, imposing time and location constraints. The evolving need for Life Long Learning (LLL) but the impossibility of attending regular courses or paying enrolment fees has led to the emergence of online modalities of instruction which cater to large numbers of potential learners who do not need to be physically in the same place to receive instruction or pay large enrolment fees. These asynchronous courses are available at different times and locations depending on the learner's physical context and so are more adaptable to the participant's life course. The aim of these courses is to align learners' needs, skills and motivations with educational contents and methodologies while allowing participants to dictate the rhythm with which they want to study and emphasize certain aspects and themes and, in this way, take charge of one's own education. One of the most utilized vehicles in this educational transformation are the Massive Open Online Courses (MOOCs). These are web-based online courses offered for learners regardless of their age, race, social, or educational status. These courses have the possibility of reaching participants in diverse settings and contexts with the only requisite, in many cases, of having an internet connection.

Table 1. Summary of the principles that constitute each of the different approaches to the paradigm of Universal Design applied to education (Adapted from Sala, *et al.*, 2014).

Terms	Universal Design for Learning	Universal Instructional Design	Universal Design for Instruction	Universal Design for Education
Principles	Provide multiple means of representation Provide multiple means of action and expression Provide multiple means of engagement	Accessible and impartial in all the parts Consistent and simple Flexible in the presentation, participation and use Explicitly presented and easily perceived Provide a support learning environment Minimize effort and requirements	Create a welcome atmosphere in class Determine the essential contents of the course Provide clear expectations and feedback Explore ways to incorporate natural support for learning Use different methods of instruction Provide different ways to demonstrate knowledge Use technology to improve learning opportunities Encourage faculty student contacts	Fair use Flexible use Intuitive and simple use Perceptible information Error tolerance Under physical effort Measures and adequate spaces Learning communities Climate of welcoming and inclusive teaching	Fair use Flexible use Intuitive and simple use Perceptible information Error tolerance Under physical effort Measures and adequate spaces
Application Centers	Center for Applied Special Technology	Georgian College Brock University University of Queens, University of Guelph	University of Minnesota	University of Connecticut University of Wisconsin	University of Washington
Main Authors	Rose & Meyer	Silver, Bouke and Strehom Bryson Palmer	Higbee	Scott, Shaw & McGuire	Burgstahler

In MOOC, it is important to carefully analyse the design and implementation of both the contents and presentations to address the different ways students learn online. This is especially true in the case of learners with Special Educational

Needs due to the constraints involved in following a course with no teacher-student interaction, or in many cases even peer to peer contact.

MOOCs have the advantage of reaching out to a global audience although it may also have the difficulty of including educational practices and approaches which may suit a certain cultural context but may be at odds with the way learners from different cultures and languages are used to using educational resources (Ke, Chávez, & Herrera 2013). Although learner-instructor interaction is an important factor in increasing completion of tasks and a positive outcome of the MOOC, currently due to the large numbers of participants enrolled in MOOC courses, or the cost both in time and personnel of this follow up, maintaining these interactions is minimal.

Phan (2018) mentioned that as in any educational program, a MOOC should also try to articulate a series of best practices which would help not only develop a better course, but also more positive participation and outcome from those participants enrolled in the course. These best practices would be:

Presentation skills: Using video presentations that convey friendliness, adequate body gestures and verbal tone, and a personalized message to all future participants.

Strong content: A sound and consistent content, directly related to the ends of the course with the inclusion of accessible material.

Managerial skills: Including an adequate flow of course content as consistently as possible.

Personalization: Encourage small group gatherings to offer different opportunities for peer discussions and feedback. The use of social media (facebook, twitter, *etc.*) or personalized emails could also be a way of greeting participants more involved in the learning process.

Feedback: The use of instant feedback, such as notifications of responses to threads in which a learner posts, or at least to the exercises completed by the learners.

Fostering learner-centred interaction: Allow participants to search for the information they might find relevant in online discussions or threads. Each participant could decide their level of involvement and their need to seek new information which must be rapidly available.

Inclusive education arises from the idea that although people may differ in the way they learn, they are all entitled to the same equal opportunities, especially regarding gaining access to high-quality education and a supportive learning environment which takes into consideration possible Special Education Needs (SEN). As we have previously stated, within the current educational instruction the use of online courses has rapidly evolved from a novelty into the way millions of people worldwide are accessing information and developing life-long education patterns with less time and space constraints. Learners with SEN are also entitled to enrol in courses that consider certain specific needs and adapt the instruction to address this situation in a more inclusive fashion.

As a specific example of all the above mentioned, we will refer to the En-Abilities project (Erasmus + project 2017-1-ES01-KA204-038155) which has been financed by the Sepie, Servicio Español para la Internacionalización de la Educación (Spanish Service for the Internationalization of Education and the European Union). This is a project implemented from September 2017 until February 2020 with partners from Ireland, Portugal, Romania Serbia and Spain. The aim of the project is to develop a comprehensive online autonomous learning tool which facilitates that people with Special Educational Needs may be able to communicate in a foreign language, in this case, English. The main reason for the project is to allow people in situations of marginalization and exclusion (socially and from the labour market) to be able to acquire knowledge in a specific tool (English) that may help their inclusion with society increasing the employability and social participation of these learners.

Recommendation 2006/962/EC of the European Parliament and Council of December 18th, 2006 resulted in the European Framework for Key Competences for Lifelong Learning, where communication in foreign languages is defined as one of the 8 lifelong learning key-competences:

1. Communication in the mother tongue;
2. Communication in foreign languages;
3. Mathematical competence and basic competences in science and technology;
4. Digital competence;
5. Learning to learn;
6. Social and civic competences;
7. Sense of initiative and entrepreneurship; and
8. Cultural awareness and expression.

Competences are defined as a combination of knowledge, skills and attitudes that all individuals need for personal fulfilment and development, active citizenship, social inclusion and employment. All the key competences are defined as equally important since they contribute to a successful life for the individual in what is considered nowadays a knowledge society. Regarding the specific competence of communication in a foreign language, the definition provided in the Recommendation states as follows:

Communication in foreign languages broadly shares the main skill dimensions of communication in the mother tongue: it is based on the ability to understand, express and interpret concepts, thoughts, feelings, facts and opinions in both oral and written form (listening, speaking, reading and writing) in an appropriate range of societal and cultural contexts (in education and training, work, home and leisure) according to one's wants or needs. Communication in foreign languages also calls for skills such as mediation and intercultural understanding. An individual's level of proficiency will vary between the four dimensions (listening, speaking, reading and writing) and between the different languages, and according to that individual's social and cultural background, environment, needs and/or interests.

The essential knowledge, skills and attitudes related to this competence are also explained in the recommendation:

Competence in foreign languages requires knowledge of vocabulary and functional grammar and an awareness of the main types of verbal interaction and registers of language. Knowledge of societal conventions and the cultural aspect and variability of languages is important.

Essential skills for communication in foreign languages consist of the ability to understand spoken messages, to initiate, sustain and conclude conversations and to read, understand and produce texts appropriate to the individual's needs. Individuals should also be able to use aids appropriately and learn languages also informally as part of lifelong learning. A positive attitude involves the appreciation of cultural diversity and an interest and curiosity in languages and intercultural communication.

Especially due to its worldwide importance and uses, the knowledge and acquisition of English language skills is deemed of great importance in our societies. All people, including people with disabilities, should have the opportunity of accessing training skills that suit their abilities and interests, but that also are relevant for the labor market (International Labor Office Skills and Employability Department and the Government of Flanders, 2007). In other words, people with SEN should be offered the same opportunities to receive training that is relevant to the latest trends in the market and to apply to available job opportunities. In this sense knowledge of the English language has become a much-required skill in contemporary societies. Currently, there are scarce online tools for learning English which accomplishes the main European guidelines regarding accessibility and Design4All.

Learning a foreign language is an opportunity that provides students with the possibility to investigate their own language and culture, compare them with additional languages and cultures, acquire communication skills in another language, critically think about the world that they live in and develop acceptance of others (Wight 2015). However, this kind of knowledge is sometimes considered less essential for people with disabilities as in "*learning foreign languages is too difficult, thus don't impose even more work on this learner, or this group of learners*" (European Commission, 2005, p. 1). This has led to a situation in which many students with disabilities cannot benefit from this opportunity and are exempted during their education of learning languages. In this sense, Sparks (2009, p. 18) defends the right to foreign language learning for this population and states that students with disabilities should "*be enrolled in foreign language courses and provided with appropriate teaching methods and instruction accommodations so that they can be successful in these classes*".

Access to an inclusive and quality education remains elusive for many people with disabilities. Adequate access should support disabled people participating fully in society and improving their quality of life. To obtain this goal, learning resources must be adapted to the needs, capacities and expectations of people with disabilities. The "one size fits all" model for language learning does not consider the specific needs of people with disabilities, and so a more inclusive program derived from knowledge obtained from studies in education conducted with people at risk of social exclusion, disabilities, or universal design for education must be created and tested with learners within these groups or collectivities.

This tool http://en-abilities.eu/the-tool/ has been devised as a MOOC course comprising units referring to the A1, A2 and B1 Common European Framework of Reference (CEFR) regarding language acquisition. These levels are deemed relevant because they consist of the basic knowledge a student should have of a foreign language (A1 and A2), and the first stage of the independent level of language acquisition (B1).

Common European Framework of Reference for Languages

The European Union has specifically described "*what language learners need to learn in order to use a language for communication and what knowledge and skills they have to develop so as to be able to act effectively*" (Council of Europe 2015, p. 1). Having a framework of reference allows institutions to share common ground for the description of objectives, content and methods, which enhances the transparency of courses and qualifications. According to this framework, reference levels are divided into the following categories: proficient user (C2 and C1), independent user (B2 and B1) and basic user (A2 and A1). For each level, competence related to understanding (listening and reading), speaking (spoken interaction and spoken production), and writing is assessed. The contents that are included within each level are briefly explained in Table **2** (Council of Europe 2015, p. 33-34):

Table 2. English language levels (CEFR).

Level	Contents
Level A1 (Breakthrough)	This is the lowest level of generative language use. The learner can interact in a simple way, ask and answer simple questions about themselves, where they live, people they know, and things they have, initiate and respond to simple statements in areas of immediate need or on very familiar topics, rather than relying purely on a very finite rehearsed, lexically organized repertoire of situation-specific phrases.
Level A2	The majority of descriptors stating social functions are found in this level, like use of simple everyday polite forms of greeting and address; ask how they are and react to news; handle very short social exchanges; ask and answer questions about what they do at work and in spare time; make and respond to invitations; discuss what to do, where to go and make arrangements to meet; make and accept offers.
Level B1	It is considered the threshold level for a visitor to a foreign country. It includes two features. First, the ability to maintain interaction and get across what you want to in a range of contexts. For example: generally follow the main points of extended discussion around him/her, provided speech is clearly articulated in standard dialect; give or seek personal views and opinions in an informal discussion with friends; express the main point he/she wants to make comprehensibly; exploit a wide range of simple language flexibly to express much of what he or she wants to; maintain a conversation or discussion but may sometimes be difficult to follow when trying to say exactly what he/she would like to; keep going comprehensibly, even though pausing for grammatical and lexical planning and repair is very evident, especially in longer stretches of free production. The second feature is the ability to cope flexibly with problems in everyday life, for example, cope with less routine situations on public transport; deal with most situations likely to arise when making travel arrangements through an agent or when actually travelling; enter unprepared into conversations on familiar topics; make a complaint; take some initiatives in an interview/consultation (*e.g.* to bring up a new subject) but is very dependent on interviewer in the interaction; ask someone to clarify or elaborate what they have just said.
Level B2	This level focuses on effective argument and being aware of your language mistakes.
Level C1	This level is labelled as Effective Operational Proficiency. It is characterized by good access to a broad range of language, which allows fluent, spontaneous communication.
Level C2	This level is considered "Mastery" and is characterized by a degree of precision, appropriateness and ease with the language which typifies the speech of those who have been highly successful learners.

Regarding students with disabilities, this document encourages their learning of a foreign language and specifically mentions what has been developed to overcome difficulties derived from working with texts (Council of Europe, 2015, p. 94):

"Devices ranging from simple hearing aids to eye-operated computer speech synthesizers have been developed to overcome even the most severe sensory and motor difficulties, whilst the use of appropriate methods and strategies has enabled young people with learning difficulties to achieve worthwhile foreign language learning objectives with remarkable success. Lip-reading, the exploitation of residual hearing and phonetic training have enabled the severely deaf to achieve a high level of speech communication in a second or foreign language. Given the necessary determination and encouragement, human beings have an extraordinary capacity to overcome obstacles to communication and the production and understanding of texts".

Considering all these ideas, the main objectives of the En-Abilities tool are to:

- Develop a Virtual Learning Environment (VLE) that facilitates autonomous language learning for adult students with Special Educational Needs (SEN) in formal and non-formal settings.
- Create a series of validated practical guidelines with evidence-based methodologies.
- Create practical guidelines for Information and Communication Technology (ICT) and software developers and pedagogical guidelines for teachers.

This design is deemed innovative because it will comprise a sequenced meaningful learning process suitable for being adapted to each student by means of adjusting the tool to several Universal Design requirements, allowing people to access information from many different devices and displaying information in an appropriate layout.

As a result of the project, a series of outputs and documents will be developed which will lead to:

The creation of personalised pathways for learning languages according to students' capacities and adapted to the Spanish, Irish, Italian, Serbian, Portuguese and Romanian contexts.

- A MOOC for encouraging the autonomous English learning of adults with SEN in formal and non-formal education settings.
- A compilation of accessible resources for learning English adapted to the capacities of adult students with SEN.
- A series of technical and pedagogical guidelines on Universal Design for learning language solutions addressed to ICT/software developers and educational professionals to adapt or create solutions to language learning for adult students with SEN.

Nevertheless, before we create a MOOC like this, it is important to undergo a needs assessment evaluation in order to know the possible language experience and knowledge of learners with SEN and to understand the attitudes, beliefs and experience of English language teachers.

First, we need to coherently test if this level of English proficiency is adequate for learners with SEN. To do so we conducted a series of levelling tests in Spain. A total of 15 participants took part in the study. Two of them presented Down syndrome, 2 presented Asperger syndrome, and the rest of the learners presented different levels of intellectual disabilities. As for completed studies, they had mostly finished primary studies (13 participants) and secondary studies (2 participants). By using a standardized English language placement test results showed that participants mostly had an English level equivalent to elementary (A1 to A2), varying from beginner (A1) to intermediate (B1). These results are similar to those found using the same placement test in Portugal, Romania and Serbia with over 50 individuals with different types of SEN (mild intellectual disability, visual impairment, and motor disability among others). Although this is not a representative sample of learners with SEN, the comparison, and the replicability of results, allow us to work with the idea that people with SEN do have a basic knowledge of English as a second language, but that if the course is to be useful and adapted to real-life situations, the MOOC must address the current abilities and competencies of the participants with the aim of improving these in order to obtain at least a B1 English level in which a person is defined as having the sufficient knowledge and skills to start being independent in the use of this second language.

Second, as Sharma, Fori & Loreman (2008) noted, the beliefs, knowledge, skills and attitudes a teacher may have regarding the general idea of inclusion in education, and the specific target groups that come to mind when thinking about inclusion have a relevant influence in both the eagerness, maintenance or ability to include diverse educational patterns within their classroom. Teachers who share more positive attitudes towards inclusion are more prone to using different and novel teaching strategies to accommodate students' individual differences (Forlin, 2010). In this sense, the preservice preparation and attitudes of the teachers of English as a second language in general and specifically those related to students with Special Education Needs (SEN), must be addressed and reviewed before commencing a new educational program. If the aim is for teachers to use, and supervise, any autonomous learning program we must understand their knowledge and skills in language teaching and their view of students with SEN. Language is both the content and medium for language acquisition and so must be optimized for understanding by modifying the necessary elements to make it more comprehensible for students who may not have direct interaction with teachers, by developing materials and accommodating them to the needs of online students with SEN in order to create new learning strategies that ease learning processes.

In 2002, Avramidis & Norwich reviewed teachers' attitudes towards the inclusion of children with SEN in mainstream school. Results showed that although attitudes were generally positive there was no acceptance of total inclusion. These attitudes towards inclusion were influenced by a) child- related variables such as the nature and severity of the disability. They were more willing to accept less severe disabled students, especially if they had physical or sensory problems instead of cognitive and emotional-behavioural disabilities; b) environment-related variables such as availability of physical and human support, and c) less by teacher-related variables such as gender, age, years of teaching, contact with disabled people and personality factors.

Although the competence of communication in foreign languages may seem quite straightforward, and the competence, skills and knowledge related to it seem to be obvious content for all teachers involved in foreign language teaching when it comes to teaching adult students with disabilities, the challenges teachers need to face cannot be easily overcome due to lack of training and knowledge in this respect. In fact, we can state that at present, there is no tool for learning English that meets the requirements set out in the main European guidelines on accessibility and design for all. Therefore, more attention needs to be paid to how to improve this situation since even in the European strategy for disability 2010-2020 in the section on raising awareness there is a direct reference to the need for particular attention towards the accessibility of materials and information channels and to promoting awareness of 'design for all' approaches to products, services and environments. Considering the EU Recommendation from 2006 and the European strategy for disability 2010-2020, the EN-ABILITIES project specifically addresses current shortcomings regarding foreign language learning for adult with disabilities through the development of a Virtual Learning Environment that aims to cover a need for lifelong training for a group at risk of exclusion if they are not given a real equality of opportunity.

Although a Virtual Learning Environment such as a MOOC is created to allow autonomous learning by students, it is also a tool which may be used by teachers of English as a foreign language, or other educators, as an accompanying tool to their own courses. As such it is important to understand that as Kormos & Nijakowska (2017) state many teachers lack appropriate training in inclusive practices that allow them to respond to learner needs in diverse settings, helping all students participate and feel a part of the complete learning process. It is important to understand the ideas, attitudes and needs of teachers in order to support their language teaching by giving them a MOOC tool which, although may be used autonomously by students under no direct supervision, may also bear in mind the knowledge and expectations of English language teachers.

In the En-Abilities project, a total of 114 English language teachers from Spain (n=54) and Portugal (n=60) answered a questionnaire regarding their experience of teaching people with disabilities and their attitudes towards this teaching process. The mean age of the teachers was 45.23 years with a standard deviation of 7.85. 44 teachers were men (38.6%) and 70 women (61.4%). Regarding their level of expertise in English 70.2% (n=80) stated that their knowledge was equivalent to a C2 level, whilst another 21.9% (n= 25) stated that it was C1. 86% of the teachers stated that they had been teaching English for 10 or more years, and 67% had taught for over 15 years. These results show that the participants were both proficient as English language teachers and had been employed as such for a considerable amount of time. Since these teachers could be considered as expert teachers in English as a second language, we were interested in knowing if they had ever taught learners with SEN. An important number of teachers stated that depending on the need they never or rarely taught people with SEN (from 42.1% to 79.8%). The less frequent participants with which the teachers interacted in their job were people with autism (79.8%), visual impairments (78.9%), physical (74.6%) and hearing impairments (72.8%). The most frequent interaction groups were learners with dyslexia (30.7% of teachers stated that they taught frequently or very frequently), and intellectual impairments (21.9%).

As for the opinion regarding if people with SEN should learn English, teachers' attitudes were tested using a Likert scale in which 1 indicated complete disagreement and 5 complete agreement with the given assumption. Teachers believe that all people must learn English (in every case over 50%), but there are differences when dealing with specific disabilities.

Table **3** shows the mean and the standard deviation of the attitudes towards the different types of disabilities.

Participants obtained high scores in positive attitudes toward learning English in all the disabilities. However, there were more positive attitude towards people with physical, visual and hearing disabilities, and more negative attitude towards the group of people with severe intellectual disability brain injury or neurological disorders. In general, the participating teachers do not doubt that all students (regardless of their disability) must learn English as a foreign language, but there is more acceptance when it is related to a physical or sensory disability, not agreeing so much when it refers to an intellectual disability with serious repercussions in the student's daily life. These results confirm Avramidis & Norwich's (2002) results in that attitudes may be positive, but more so depending on the specific disability.

Table 3. Participants' attitudes toward learning English in the population of persons with different types of disabilities.

Type of disability	M	SD
1. Delayed speech and language development	4.02	1.07
2. Specific learning disabilities	4.08	1.01
3. Mild intellectual disability	4.12	0.90
4. Severe forms of intellectual disability	3.39	1.29
5. ADHD	4.15	1.02
6. Visual impairment	4.57	0.72
7. Hearing impairment	4.27	0.97
8. Physical disabilities	4.73	0.58
9. Mental disorders	3.77	1.15
10. Behavioural disorders	4.18	1.01
11. Brain injury/neurological disorders	3.55	1.27
12. Autism spectrum disorder	4.03	1.11

Another important aspect related to teachers' interaction with learners with SEN is how they adapt their teaching methods to students with special needs. The Portuguese and Spanish participants in this study stated that they mostly adapted and simplified the program, teaching methods and tasks. For instance, they divided tasks into smaller, simpler steps, requiring students with disabilities to do only tasks which they found interesting or which were related to tasks they had recently done. Also, they thought that it was very important to offer extra material or different activities (for example manipulative activities or handing out materials beforehand of each lesson). Teachers also used accommodations such as giving extended time to complete a task. Some teachers paid special attention to students with SEN (*e.g.* they approached these students more frequently), while some emphasized adapting teaching materials and the learning environment (*e.g.* a privileged seat for a student with SEN). They also recognized the significance of adapting the way content was presented, and thus emphasized using visual support (pictures and drawings) and multimodal teaching approach (presenting the content in a visual, auditory and tactile-kinaesthetic way).

These teachers also paid great attention to if learners had correctly understood the content of each lesson. English language teachers frequently checked whether learners with SEN understood the instructions, and repeated significant information, encouraging self-correction before instructional correction.

Teachers involved in the study were aware of the need to adapt teaching methods for persons with SEN, and they recognized many different possible strategies. In sum results show that their knowledge on educational needs of students with SEN is significant, but some assumptions regarding the possibility of teaching English to students with certain disabilities must be addressed and contents and methods must be structured in a way (*i.e.* by means of specific handouts and textbooks for teachers which address SEN and universal design) which may help teachers' and learners obtain maximum reward from their efforts and learning process.

ACCOMMODATIONS FOR ENGLISH LEARNERS WITH SEN

As stated before, English language teachers, students, pedagogues, ICT professionals and all other professionals and people involved in developing educational programs for people with SEN must know how to accommodate their contents to the need for inclusive education. As Kormos (2017) stated, learners with SEN not only face native language processing problems but also difficulties acquiring the knowledge and ability to interact successfully in additional languages. These learners need to be taught using inclusive methodologies and contents which enable them to achieve an adequate level of language acquisition reflecting the individual differences in learners.

While constructing the En-Abilities project, we have contacted over 150 English language teachers, over 50 English language students with SEN, teachers and pedagogues who work with learners with SEN, teachers who themselves have SEN, organizations, associations and other professionals so that they could put forward, based on their expertise and personal experiences, a series of accommodations which may help the MOOC reach out to a larger numbers of potential learners. The educational tool must be fully inclusive and based on the needs of the learners, adapting contents and methodologies to these participants and not the other way around. Apart from obviously fully complying with W3C accessibility guidelines (https://www.w3.org/standards/webdesign/accessibility), some of the most relevant accommodations included within the En-Abilities MOOC are:

1.- Although it might seem quite conspicuous, the first accommodation is to include a MOOC tutorial written in accessible language to help students engage in the course. This tutorial should be written both in English and the native language due to the level of English participants have at the beginning of the course.
2.- Correctly explain what the student must do (written text, spoken text, both in English and native language), especially for the first units. Answering options need to be explicit (being very precise regarding what the learner must do to

answer). The way one must answer questions must be adapted to different educational needs (*i.e.* Click and dragging is hard for motor and visual disabilities. It must be made easier by increasing sensitivity of the boxes or not used).

3.- There should be a gradual decrease in the use of native language and include examples to allow the learner to understand how it must be answered correctly. The inclusion of video messages and examples will help learners understand the exact nature of the lesson and examples. The inclusion of people with disabilities in these videos will also help learners identify situations depicted in the example with less problems.

4.- Typeface should be Sans Serif and at least use a 14-point font. It is important to delete bold typeface from the text. Alternative text, audio-descriptions and explanations should be included both in English and native language.

5.- Inclusion of alternative text (both written and spoken). We must allow page readers such as JAWS and page augmenters such as Zoomtext to be used with the MOOC lesson

- Authors such as Fernández-Portero (2018) have stated that students with functional diversity should be presented all possible information not only in English but also in their native language.
- There should be an option for this alternative text to appear or not depending on the needs of the participant.
- Create text which is simple and easy to understand. It must include details which clearly exemplify the images or concepts (*i.e.* If we present a chef, state that the person *"Works in a restaurant, wears a hat and uses a knife";* For a doctor: *"Works in a hospital and cures disease and illness"*).

Prepare the material so that screen readers can be used and include an audio for each exercise.

6.- Include a button which may change the image from colour to black and white (to help people with visual impairment).

7.- Feedback should be substantive and informative, not comparative, competitive or confrontative (*i.e* Great!!!, Try again!! Nearly there!!!)

8.- Examples must not be culturally dependent. All images, pictures and sound bites should have a meaning that can be easily comprehensible for students in different parts of the world. For instance, there should be few references to culturally specific issues such as religious holidays, specific large population gatherings, or other examples that need cultural clarification. This must be especially obvious in the first lessons of any unit, and these differences should only appear after a process of gradually getting from the more general and global (shared) view of daily interactions to the more particular interactions of specific cultures which then should be addressed in units specifically designed to analyse cultural similarities and differences.

9.- Students must be able to relate their native language to what they are learning in English. The possibility of referencing vocabulary written or spoken in English to written and oral sentences in the native language is a way of enhancing bilingualism and making students more comfortable with the lessons in an autonomous setting. It should be used as an early resource to assist and comfort students but not applied in all instances to develop an urge for students to use other available resources to answer some doubts.

10.- The inclusion of gender-neutral images and pictures, non-stereotypical gender roles, incorporating images of people with disabilities performing everyday activities and interactions is viewed to normalize a more inclusive worldview through exposure and not targeted instruction. Whenever possible the use of real-life photographs would be appropriate because it facilitates the recognition of a person or a job and also helps to not infantilize participants. The main aim of a MOOC should be to help students learn English in an autonomous way. Although the content and attractiveness of the units are a fundamental aspect of the program, inclusiveness and universal design are as important because by addressing everyday situations with the presence of certain target groups which would normally not be included within the examples of the program, the cosmovision of future students will be broadened normalizing situations and learning processes which may be seen for many as somewhat alien in current educational programs.

CONCLUSION AND DISCUSSION

Inclusion is one of the most spoken words in the world. It is politically correct to address the need to embrace human diversity and to include it in society. But to what extent such inclusion is effectively implemented? We live in a globalized society where large borders no longer exist. Markets and jobs dissipate geographical boundaries and assume international characteristics. Much of life is spent online communicating. Communication is assumed as the foundation of society and, consequently, of inclusion in different societal contexts. Those who do not communicate effectively find barriers and are at a disadvantage compared to others. English is assumed as a universal language conveyed in science, politics and even in everyday life when different nationalities meet. The inclusion of persons with disabilities in an international context is often undervalued because a person with special needs is not expected to internationalize. However, people with disabilities migrate, work from a distance and relate to other nationalities in terms of work, where English is often the bridge. There is a need to promote the learning of English in a contemporary way, in order to reach as many people as possible. In this context, online learning, through MOOCs, is widespread.

However, it is necessary to safeguard the validity and effectiveness of the teaching and learning process, and above all ensure accessibility for people with functional limitations. It is within this scope that the EN-ABILITIES Project arises. As a result of European cooperation, it seeks to deliver a viable and effective option for learning English by non-native speakers with disabilities and Special Educational Needs. It is based on an effective survey of the needs of potential students and the perspective of those who teach English to people with disabilities. This project, based on the guidelines of Universal Design for Learning, aims to produce not only an online course, but also practical guides and validated content for learning English by people with disabilities in the European world.

CONSENT FOR PUBLICATION

Not applicable.

CONFLICT OF INTEREST

The author confirms that this chapter contents have no conflict of interest.

ACKNOWLEDGEMENTS

The authors acknowledge the ERASMUS + Programme for research funding of the project with the reference 2017-1-ES01-KA201-038155. This publication reflects the views only of the authors, and the Commission cannot be held responsible for any use which may be made of the information contained therein.

REFERENCES

Avramidis, E., Norwich, B. (2002). Teachers' attitudes towards integration/inclusion: A review of the literature. *Eur. J. Spec. Needs Educ., 17*, 129-147.

Council of Europe. (2015). *Common European Framework of Reference of Languages: Learning, teaching, assessment.* https://rm.coe.int/1680459f97

European Commission. (2005). *Special Education Needs in Europe. The Teaching & Learning of Languages.* http://tictc.cti.gr/documents/doc647_en.pdf

European Disability Strategy 2010-2020. *A Renewed Commitment to a Barrier-Free Europe.* https://eur-lex.europa.eu/LexUriServ/LexUriServ.do?uri=COM:2010:0636:FIN:en:PDF

Fernández Portero, I. (2018). Diseño universal para el aprendizaje de idiomas en personas con diversidad funcional. (Universal design for learning languages in people with functional diversity). *Revista de Educación Inclusiva, 11*(1), 251-266.

Forlin, C. (2010). Re-framing teacher education for inclusion.*Teacher Education for Inclusion: Changing Paradigms and Innovative Approaches.* (pp. 3-10). Abingdon: Routledge. [http://dx.doi.org/10.4324/9780203850879]

Government of Spain. (2003). Ley 51/2003, de 2 de diciembre, de igualdad de oportunidades, no discriminación y accesibilidad universal de las personas con discapacidad.

Government of Spain. (2007a). Ley Orgánica 4/2007, de 12 de abril, por la que se modifica la Ley Orgánica 6/2001, de 21 de diciembre, de Universidades. *BOE, 89*, 16241-16260.

Government of Spain. (2007b). Real Decreto 1393/2007, de 29 de octubre, por el que se establece la ordenación de las enseñanzas universitarias oficiales.

Government of Spain. (2013a). Ley Orgánica 8/2013, de 9 de diciembre, para la mejora de la calidad educativa.

Government of Spain. (2013b). Real Decreto Legislativo 1/2013, de 29 de noviembre, por el que se aprueba el Texto Refundido de la Ley General de derechos de las personas con discapacidad y de su inclusión social.

International Labor Office Skills and Employability Department and the Government of Flanders. (2007). *Strategies for Skills Acquisition and Work for Persons with Disability in Southern Africa Zambia.* [Online at http://www.ilo.org/wcmsp5/groups/public/@ed_emp/@ifp_skills/documents/publication/wcms_107784.pdf , retrieved on November 7th 2018. International Organization for Standardization. (1998). *Guidance on usability ISO 9241-11.*

Iwarsson, S., Ståhl, A. (2003). Accessibility, usability and universal design--positioning and definition of concepts describing person-environment relationships. *Disabil. Rehabil., 25*(2), 57-66.
[http://dx.doi.org/10.1080/dre.25.2.57.66] [PMID: 12554380]

Ke, F., Chávez, A.F., Herrera, F. (2013). *Web-based Teaching and Learning Across Culture and Age.* New York: Springer.
[http://dx.doi.org/10.1007/978-1-4614-0863-5]

Kormos, J. (2017). *The Second Language Learning Process of Students with Specific Learning Difficulties.* New York: Routledge.

Kormos, J., Nijakowska, J. (2017). Inclusive practices in teaching students with dyslexia: Second language teachers' concerns, attitudes and self-efficacy beliefs on a massive open online learning course. *Teach. Teach. Educ., 68*, 30-41.
[http://dx.doi.org/10.1016/j.tate.2017.08.005]

Phan, T. (2018). Instructional strategies that respond to global learners' needs in massive open online courses. *Online Learn., 22*(2), 95-118.
[http://dx.doi.org/10.24059/olj.v22i2.1160]

Preiser, W., Ostrosff, E. (2001). *Universal Design Handbook* (1st ed.). New York: McGraw Hill.

Preiser, W., Smith, K.H. (2011). Introduction.*Universal Design Handobook.* McGraw Hill.

Real Patronato sobre Discapacidad (Ed.). (2011). *Estrategia sobre discapacidad 2012 - 2020.* (Strategy towards disability 2012-2020. Madrid. Recommendation of the European Parliament and of the Council of 18 December 2006 on key competences for lifelong learning (2006/962/EC) https://eur-lex.europa.eu/lega--content/EN/TXT/?uri=celex%3A32006H0962

Sala, I., Sánchez, S., Giné, C., Díez, E. (2014). Análisis de los distintos enfoques del paradigma del diseño universal aplicado a la educación. (Analysis of the different perspectives on universal design paradigm applied to eduaction). *Revista Iberoamericana de Educación Inclusiva, 8*(1), 143-152.

Sánchez, S., Díez, E., Martín, R.Á. (2015). El diseño universal como medio para atender a la diversidad en la educación. Una revisión de casos de éxito en la universidad. (Universal design as a way to deal with diversity in eduaction. A review of success examples in the university). *Contextos Educativos. Revista de Educación, 19*, 121-131.https://publicaciones.unirioja.es/ojs/index.php/contextos/article/view/2752

Sharma, U., Forlin, C., Loreman, T. (2008). Impact of training on pre-service teachers' attitudes and concerns about inclusive education and sentiments about persons with disabilities. *Disabil. Soc., 23*(7), 773-785.
[http://dx.doi.org/10.1080/09687590802469271]

Sparks, R.L. (2009). If you don't know where you're going, you'll wind up somewhere else: The case of foreign language learning disability. *Foreign Lang. Ann., 42*, 7-26.

[http://dx.doi.org/10.1111/j.1944-9720.2009.01005.x]

Story, M.F. (2011). The principles of Universal Design. *Universal Design Handobook.* (2nd ed.). New York: McGraw Hill.

Webb, K.K., Hoover, J. (2015). Universal design for learning (UDL) in the academic library: A methodology for mapping multiple means of representation in library tutorials. *Coll. Res. Libr., 76*(4), 537-553. [http://dx.doi.org/10.5860/crl.76.4.537]

Webb, J., Williams, B.T., Smith, K.H. (2011). Redefining Design and Disability: A person-environment fit model. *Universal Design Handobook.* (2nd ed.). New York: McGraw Hill.

Wight, M.C. (2015). Students with learning disabilities in the foreign language learning environment and the practice of exemption. *Foreign Lang. Ann., 48*(1), 39-55. [http://dx.doi.org/10.1111/flan.12122]

Zolkowska, T., Kasior-Szerszen, I., Blaszkiewicz, I. (2002). European union policy toward people with disabilities. *Disabil. Stud. Q., 22*(4), 217-224. [http://dx.doi.org/10.18061/dsq.v22i4.387]

CHAPTER 4

The Daily Life´s Routines of Children with Disabilities

Helena Mesquita[1,*], João Serrano[2], Samuel Honório[2], Marco Batista[2] and **Jaime Ribeiro[3]**

[1] *Instituto Politécnico de Castelo Branco/Centro Interdisciplinar de Ciências Sociais (CICS.NOVA)/Sport, Health & Exercise Reseach Unit (SHERU), Portugal*

[2] *Sport, Health & Exercise Reseach Unit (SHERU)/Instituto Politécnico de Castelo Branco, Portugal*

[3] *School of Health Sciences & ciTechCare - Center for Innovative Care and Health Technology, Polytechnic of Leiria, Portugal/CIDTFF - Research Centre on Didactics and Technology in the Education of Trainers - University of Aveiro, Portugal*

Abstract: The objective of this research is to know the activities, the routes, the places visited and the obstacles identified in daily life routines of children/youth with disabilities, living in urban environments, during the time in which they are off the school period. In methodological terms, we used as instruments of study an anamnesis fact sheet and a routine diary that was completed by the parents together with the child/youth, an Individual Educational Plans (IEP) and a semi-structured narrative interview. Eight subjects between the ages of 9 and 15, all with different pathologies, were part of the study. The study was exploratory, descriptive and analytical. The results demonstrated that the subjects are supported in their routines by their parents and other relatives. Weekly out-of-school routines are primarily focused in the home (meaningful and important place) with activities classified mostly as sedentary ones in which they use little materials and, in the places, where they perform specific activities (Therapies, Tutoring, Music Conservatory and Catechism). The age and pathologies associated with each subject are factors that influence autonomy and independence of mobility. They visited few places and did so mainly in the company of family members. The main obstacles encountered in the routes performed are closely related to their pathology, showing difficulties in interacting with their peers. We conclude that the children/young people who participated in the study engaged in few activities and these were mostly in the home and sedentary. They visit few places, have poor independence of mobility, and interact poorly with others.

Keywords: Activities, Autonomy, Children, Disability, Mobility, Movement, Objects and subjects, Obstacles, Physical activity, Places frequented, Routes,

---

[*] **Corresponding author Helena Mesquita:** Instituto Politécnico de Castelo Branco/Centro Interdisciplinar de Ciências Sociais (CICS.NOVA)/Sport, Health & Exercise Reseach Unit (SHERU), Portugal; Tel: +351 272 339 100; E-mail: hmesquita@ipcb.pt

Routines of daily living, Time spent in activities, Travelling, Urban, Young people.

INTRODUCTION

The contemporary world is undergoing rapid and profound socio-economic transformations (development of the economy, social mobility, new forms of employment, new qualitative and quantitative forms of unemployment ...), family and individual, as well as in the system of values and norms that are associated with it, and also at the level of science and technology. In a society that is constantly evolving and transforming, people's life routines are being influenced by these changes that have a strong impact on their quality of life.

When we talk about daily routines and the quality of life of people with disabilities, considering the current world and its social organization, we are looking at a very particular minority of the population that should not be neglected. in an inclusive society.

According to the World Health Organization (2011), it is estimated that today there are more than 650 million people with disabilities that is about 16% of the total population (ranging from 12% in the more developed countries to 18% in the developed countries). In Europe, there are around 40 million people with disabilities and in Portugal, around 634,408, which corresponds to 6.1% of the resident population (Freire, 2010).

The fact that they have some type of long-term physical, mental, intellectual or sensorial impediment (Santos, 2016) should not be an obstructive condition of rights of full participation on equal terms with the rest of society as defined in 2007 in the Convention on the Rights of Persons with Disabilities. Greguol (2017) states that in order to determine public policies that allow the promotion of the full social inclusion of people with disabilities in different activities, it is necessary to know the reality in different countries. At present there is still an acute shortage of information on the needs of these populations, be it on part of the family, the school and society, which translates into the lack of adequate incentives for the development of their potentialities (Greguol, Gobbi & Carraro, 2013). There is also a shortage of studies on life routines, lifestyles and quality of life of people with some type of disability (Interdonato & Greguol, 2011). In order to contribute to the development in this area of study, it was our objective to know the activities, the routes, the places attended and the obstacles identified in the routines of daily life of the children/young people with a deficiency condition, living in urban areas, during the time they are off school.

Routines and Activities of People with Disabilities

When we speak of routine, it is important to clarify the concept. Santos (2016, p.3) tells us that the word "routine" is defined in the Priberam Portuguese Dictionary tas "a constant practice, habit of always doing something in the same way or sequence of instructions or steps in the realization of a task or activity".

A "daily routine" according to Pereira (2014) refers to the framing of various daily tasks or events contextualized in learning, it is related to a daily succession of flexible events, in space and time. Pinto (1995) states that routines are fundamental dimensions of everyday life because they intervene significantly in the temporal and spatial structure of everyday life. In the same way, it is said that "both the common meaning of the concept of routine and its etymology pervades the idea of repetition, habit, wheel, vicious circle" (Brandão, Gonçalves & Medeiros, 2006: 25).

The experience of a differentiated routine with respect to the contexts can be a facilitating element of this construction process. However, if the multiple and differentiated routines are not integrated into the life-style of each adolescent and in a safe and responsive family environment, these may constitute a risk factor. The family, as a context of development and socialization with an educational role, can establish the borderline between the risk and the development potential of the contexts frequented by adolescents in the course of their daily routines (Barbosa-Ducharne, Cruz, Marinho & Large, 2012). Craidy and Kaercher (2001) argue that it is necessary to organize routines considering biological needs (such as rest, food, hygiene and age), psychological needs (individual differences) and social and historical needs (with regards to culture and lifestyle). Mahoney, Harris, and Eccles (2006) also point out that the way children and adolescents use time, in particular, time away from school, has consequences for their development. Hohmann and Weikart (2011) and Pereira (2014) argue that organizing the routine allows children to anticipate what will happen next, giving them a great sense of control over what they do at any given moment, providing feelings of greater security and autonomy. The daily routines provide children with security and knowledge regarding the activities that surround them, allowing for their development and cognitive evolution. However, Folque (2014) says that there are situations in which these routines must be modified to allow the realization and value of other activities that might not be foreseen and defined previously.

Routines also appear in the literature with other names. Serrano (2003) states that in addition to "routines of life" or "ways of life" there are authors who call it "lifestyles" and be something individual or group, one can speak of the lifestyle of an individual, group or culture.

From the beginning of the 21st century, several authors (Arez & Neto, 2000; Serrano, 2003; Moreno, 2009; Lopes, 2013) were concerned with the issue of lifestyles and sought to study everyday life and mobility of children and young people with no disability, in order to understand how these daily activities were structured. More recently, this line of research has awakened the curiosity of some researchers who have sought to identify behavioural and environmental factors that can also serve as potential mediators of changes in activity habits in specific subpopulations, such as those with a deficiency. Kirchner, Gerber and Smith (2008) concluded that people with disabilities tend to have fewer active lifestyles when compared with people without disabilities, being more obese and less healthy.

The assumption that regular physical activity is associated with a number of health benefits, decreasing the risk of various diseases and even reducing the overall risk of mortality (Warburton, Nicol & Bredin, 2006) or the demonstration which has a positive impact on several cognitive and emotional parameters and is associated with a lower risk of cognitive decline and dementia (Marmeleira, Laranjo, Marques & Pereira, 2014), also led different authors to study the relationship of this activity in the life routines of individuals with disability. The authors cited add that studies show that the level of physical activity of people with disabilities in their routines of life is much lower than that of the general population, also explained by the scarcity of structured activities. Different authors (Rimmer, Riley, Wang, Rauworth & Jurkowski, 2004) have developed studies with people with visual impairment concluding that the physical activity on the part of this population can be due to the architectural barriers found in the environment, which hinder access to spaces of people's interest and also to personal barriers (motivation, fears, need for support from third parties ...). Lee, Zhu, Ackley-Holbrook, Brower & McMurray (2014) concluded that lack of motivation may be one of the factors with the most negative impact on the practice of physical activity by people with disabilities in their routines of daily living.

Urban Mobility of People with Disabilities

According to Magalhães, Aragão & Yamashita (2013, p.3) "etymologically, the term" mobility "derives from the Latin, mobilitas (attis), which in turn derives from mobilis (e) meaning mobile (that can move). It is a term that has been modified over time and presents a variety of concepts according to the different areas of knowledge and their research interests.

The notion of mobility considers the freedom with which people can move in a certain space. Some authors (Teles, 2005; Barbosa, 2016) refer that we should look at the concept of mobility beyond the simple distance between two points, we should look at people's movements and paths considering how they are performed and the interactions that occur during them. The importance of interactions and appropriation of the urban space by the people, brings a central concern that is the need to plan spaces, so that they can be freely accessible to all segments of society without exception, since it is decisive for their physical and mental well-being (Günther 2003; Gomes & Paixão, 2013).

Urban mobility is considered sustainable, according to Gomide and Galindo (2013), when people can have universal access to the opportunities that the city offers them. This is not yet a reality today, especially for the most fragile people, such as children and people with disabilities or people with reduced mobility, who find in the cities many restrictions, obstacles and constraints. In this regard, Serrano (2003) states that, despite the importance of the independence of mobility in children's lives, a finding made by different authors in different countries (Bjorklid (Sweden), Hilmann and Adams (England), Kytta (Finland), Van der Spek and Noyon (Netherlands), Huttenmoser (Switzerland), Arez, Serrano and Neto (Portugal),observed that there are still, today, in the urban surroundings many social constraints that directly influence this autonomy aggravating limitations in the possibilities of the spatial expansion of the child, aggravating this fact when they present a condition of disability. The main constraints that are mentioned as limiting the independence of mobility are very interconnected with economic and social interests which, in turn, will interfere with the way the involvement is organized. Apolo (2010) adds that many of the obstacles encountered in the urban environment (architectural barriers) which condition mobility, are the responsibility of urban planning technicians and are located on the public thoroughfare and in its surroundings (spaces, buildings and equipment). Thus, streets with narrow pavements and sometimes damaged, lack of stairways and ramps, traffic density, disintegration and social insecurity, problems with transportation and disorderly growth are, among many other factors, those that make cities a difficult place for children and people with disabilities or with reduced mobility to travel alone in the surrounding space (Apolo, 2010).

Despite the findings, we can say that this reality has improved, the result of the concerns of many researchers with autonomy and mobility in urban environments during childhood (Serrano, 2003) and by people with reduced mobility or with disabilities (Barbosa, 2016). This special interest has resulted in the emergence of a few studies on urban planning, the quality of neighbourhoods or residential areas and their outdoor spaces, and the conclusions of which have influenced policy makers to overcome many of the constraints related to autonomy and urban mobility by these people.

We believe that the growing social awareness (high volume of awareness campaigns) and political responsibility for the mobility and accessibility of citizens with disabilities to public spaces in urban areas have contributed decisively to the improvements that have occurred in the last decades since the enactment of Decree -Law nº 650/75, of November 18, reinforced by Decree-Law no. 123/97, of May 22 and Decree-Law no. 163/2006, of August 8, related to the improvement of the standards of life for all those living in urban spaces, proposing the elimination of obstacles in paths and public spaces, collective equipment and public buildings that may constitute obstacles to mobility (Apolo, 2010).

Relevance and Purpose of the Study

The life routines of children and young people allow us to know their interrelationship with their surroundings. When we talk about children with disabilities, this knowledge becomes more important in order to contribute to an increasingly inclusive society.

The objective of this research was to know the activities, routes, sites visited and obstacles identified in the routines of the daily life of children/youth with disabilities living in an urban environment, during the time they are off the school period. So one should try to:

- Seek out what activities the children/youth do in and out of the house, the time spent doing these activities, identify who the companions are, know the materials/objects used in them and know if they imply more or less movement;

- Try to characterize the routes to reach the different places and to know the main obstacles encountered in these routes;

- Identify the places visited and know which are the most important/meaningful for children/youth in their daily routines;

Type of Study

The study is based on qualitative research modality. Actions can be better understood when they are observed in the natural environment of occurrence by analysing the data in an inductive way with the researchers interested in what is behind certain behaviours or attitudes (Bogdan & Biklen, 1994).

Considering the characteristics and objectives of the study, we opted for an exploratory, descriptive and analytical study in the field of life routines. 1) To classify it as exploratory because there are few studies on this subject, involving this population. In the justification of such studies, Selltiz, Jahoda, Deutsch &

Cook (1974, p. 59) state that they "emphasize the discovery of ideas and insights, allowing us to know the characteristics of a given reality." 2) It also assumes a descriptive character, since we intend to describe the perceptual universe of the subject who experiences an experience. Marconi & Lakatos (1996, p.20) report that these types of studies "describe a phenomenon or situation, when performed in a certain space-time, 3) It also has an analytical aspect, since it allows us to compile the available data, as detailed as possible so as to be able to analyse and understand the phenomenon better.

Methodology

Subjects and Criteria of Choice

Eight children/youth with disabilities, six males and two females, aged between 9 and 14 years old and with different types of disability, as we can observe in Table 1, were included in this study. All have spoken language so they can be heard regarding their choices, being active participants in the data collection process. Six subjects live with families and two are institutionalized.

Table 1. Characterization of subjects regarding age and type of disability.

Subjects	Age	Disability
1	9 years old	Attention and Concentration Deficit
2	12 years old	Epilepsy and Asperger Syndrome
3	14 years old	Intellectual and Developmental Difficulty
4	14 years old	Right Hemiparesis
5	11 years old	Bourneville-Pringle Syndrome (Tuberous Sclerosis)
6	13 years old	Fetal Alcohol Syndrome
7	13 years old	Mosaicism
8	11 years old	Intellectual and Developmental Difficulty

This age group was considered as a period in the life of the child that is essential for their social development. This period corresponds to a phase in which new social relationships are established, where greater balance is indicated, accepting others and themselves better. According to Chombart De Lauwe, Bonnin, Mayeur, Perrot, Soudiere (1976) it is observed that there is a better integration in the infantile group. In this period, we also talk about the first stages of adolescence, where a great advance in their conceptual thought is denoted. Despite the individual limitations of each one, this age group was also considered because the child already has a greater capacity for collaboration and communication, which facilitates the collection of information. The place of data collection was convenient because we felt that the child would feel more confident and comfortable in their environment.

Instruments

Yin (1994) recommends the use of different sources and data collection techniques in the case study, since this may be considered a diversified set of analysis topics (if different sources are used for different facts and phenomena), or obtain information from different origin converging in the same direction, allowing us to have different readings about the same phenomenon. To collect data, we used the following tools: Anamnesis form, Daily Routine Plan (DRP), Individual Educational Plans (IEP) and semi-structured narrative interview. The Anamnesis Card collected data that identified the subject, the household, pregnancy and gestation, motor and psychosocial development and some clinical data; through the IEP, it was possible to have access to the educational path and the current clinical situation and with DRP, which we built, we intend to know the activities, the objects/materials used, the paths taken, the time dedicated to several activities and the routes, the places visited, the companions and obstacles or constraints, having been filled in by the parents in the course of two weeks. The semi-structured narrative interview allowed us to collect information about the child's daily life, completing the information collected through the other tools.

Data Processing

We have chosen to organize the data collected in categories that were constructed a posteriori. As we wanted to know the activities performed by the subjects outside the school period, the school activities inside the school were not included. Eight categories were considered: **Sleep; Meals; Homework/Study**: activities carried out outside the school, (homework, study and tutoring times); **Physical activity with more Movement**: guided sports activities and sports done in clubs/associations, therapies (psychomotricity, hippotherapy, occupational therapy, physical therapy), outdoor activities (running, playing catch, hide-an--seek, walking, ...); **Physical Activity with less Movement**: play activities or "fun" activities, such as watching television, playing computer or tablet, drawing, playing with objects; activities related to housekeeping (putting the dishes in the machine, tidying the bedroom, going to the movies, playing a musical instrument, a catechesis and music conservatory); **Hygiene; Travelling:** carried out (walking, car, transport, ...); **Undetermined:** this activity was considered necessary to fill the transition periods between activities and periods without a defined activity.

RESULTS

In all the studied subjects (8), the activities performed in the house during the week are concentrated in 5 categories: Sleep, Meals, Study/Homework, Hygiene and Physical Activity with less Movement, as we can see in Table **2**.

As for the activities performed <u>outside the home</u>, there is a more marked disparity in the categories: all subjects (8) perform activities related to the categories *Physical Activity with more Movement and Travelling*. Subjects 4 and 7 also present the *Meals* category, subject 3 to the *Study/Homework* category (tutoring) and subject 6 to the *Meals and Study/Homework* (tutoring) categories, as seen in Table **3**. Subject 6 is the one which presents a greater number of activities (four) outside the home and subjects 1,2,5 and 8 with fewer activities (two).

Table 2. Activities performed in-house, during the week (weekdays and weekends).

Subjects	Activities Inside the Home				
1	Sleep	Meals	Study/Homework	Hygiene	Physical Activity with less movement
2	Sleep	Meals	Study/Homework	Hygiene	Physical Activity with less movement
3	Sleep	Meals	Study/Homework	Hygiene	Physical Activity with less movement
4	Sleep	Meals	Study/Homework	Hygiene	Physical Activity with less movement
5	Sleep	Meals	Study/Homework	Hygiene	Physical Activity with less movement
6	Sleep	Meals	Study/Homework	Hygiene	Physical Activity with less movement
7	Sleep	Meals	Study/Homework	Hygiene	Physical Activity with less movement
8	Sleep	Meals	Study/Homework	Hygiene	Physical Activity with less movement

Table 3. Activities performed outside the home, during the week (weekdays and weekends).

Subjects	Activities Outside the Home			
1	Physical Activity with more Movement	Travelling	-----	-----
2	Physical Activity with more Movement	Travelling	-----	-----
3	Physical Activity with more Movement	Travelling	Study/Homework	-----
4	Physical Activity with more Movement	Travelling	-----	Meals
5	Physical Activity with more Movement	Travelling	-----	-----
6	Physical Activity with more Movement	Travelling	Study/Homework	Meals
7	Physical Activity with more Movement	Travelling	-----	Meals
8	Physical Activity with more Movement	Travelling	-----	-----

How much time did you Spend (Average in Minutes) on the Different Activities Performed Inside and Outside the Home, During Weekdays and on Weekends?

According to Table **4**, *Sleep* was always the activity that subjects spent more time on weekdays and at the weekend. <u>On weekdays,</u> half of the subjects (1,2,4 and 6) spent more time on activities included in the *Physical Activity category with less Movement*, 3 subjects (5, 7 and 8) on *Meals* and 1 subject (3) on activities related to the *Study/Homework* category. The activity that was also dedicated a longer amount of time by subjects 1, 2, 4 and 6 was related to the category *Meals*. Subject 3 did not dedicate any time to *Physical Activities with more Movement* during the weekdays and the time dedicated to *Physical Activity with less Movement* is inferior to that dedicated to carrying out activities related to the *Study/Homework* and *Meals*, as we can see in Table **2**.

Table 4. Time spent (average in minutes) in the different activities carried out inside and outside the home, during the weekdays.

Subjects	Weekdays – Time spent (average in minutes) activities inside and outside the home					
1	Sleep (481)	Physical Activity with less Movements (168)	Meals (90)	Study/ Homework (48)	Physical Activity with more movements(24)	Hygiene (20)	Travelling (20)
2	Sleep (677)	Physical Activity with less movements.(145)	Meals (116)	Travelling(63)	Physical Activity with more movements(39)	Study/ Homework (27)	Hygiene (20)
3	Sleep (562)	Study/ Homework (162)	Meals (117)	Physical Activity with less Movement(88)	Travelling((40)	Hygiene (30)	Physical Activity with more Movement(0)
4	Sleep (594)	Physical Activity with less Movement(141)	Meals (122)	Travelling((53)	Study/ Homework (49)	Physical Activity with more Movement(48)	Hygiene (28)
5	Sleep (600)	Meals (180)	Hygiene (110)	Physical Activity with less Movement(101)	Travelling (65)	Physical Activity with more Movement(63)	Study/ Homework (35)
6	Sleep (510)	Physical Activity with less Movement(162)	Meals (144)	Physical Activity with more Movement(100)	Study/ Homework (100)	Hygiene (78)	Travelling (43)
7	Sleep (540)	Meals (185)	Physical Activity with less Movement(166)	Physical Activity with more Movement(138)	Travelling(66)	Hygiene (45)	Study/ Homework (20)

(Table 4) cont.....

Subjects	Weekdays – Time spent (average in minutes) activities inside and outside the home						
8	Sleep (600)	Meals (190)	Physical Activity with less Movement(111)	Hygiene (90)	Travelling (65)	Physical Activity with more Movement(63)	Study/Homework (35)

At weekends, all subjects spent more time on activities related to *Physical Activity with less Movement*, followed by the category *Meals* for 5 subjects and *Physical Activity with more Movement* category for the remaining subjects (three). Subjects 1, 2 and 4 did not dedicate any time to activities related to the *Physical Activity category with more Movement* over the weekend (although during the week they did) and subjects 5 and 8 did not perform activities of the category *Study /Homework*, as shown in Table **5**.

Table 5. Time spent (average in minutes) in the different activities performed inside and outside the home during the weekend.

Subjects	WEEKEND - Time spent (average in minutes) activities inside and outside the home						
1	Sleep (645)	Physical Activity with less Movement(360)	Meals (220)	Study/Homework (120)	Travelling (60)	Hygiene (25)	Physical activity with more Movement(0)
2	Sleep (708)	Physical Activity with less Movement(400)	Meals (128)	Study/Homework (120)	Hygiene (35)	Mobil/ Travelling (10)	Physical activity with more Movement(0)
3	Sleep (565)	Physical Activity with less Movement(450)	Meals (210)	Study/Homework (68)	Hygiene (48)	Physical activity (45)	Travelling (33)
4	Sleep (658)	Physical Activity with less Movement(406)	Meals (180)	Study/Homework (165)	Travelling (33)	Hygiene (30)	Physical activity with more Movement(0)
5	Sleep (775)	Physical Activity with less Movement(215)	Physical activity with more Movement(160)	Meals (135)	Hygiene (110)	Travelling (40)	Study/Homework (0)
6	Sleep (810)	Physical Activity with less Movement(398)	Physical activity with more Movement(193)	Meals (170)	Hygiene (65)	Study/Homework (20)	Travelling (10)
7	Sleep (585)	Physical Activity with less Movement(393)	Meals (218)	Physical activity with more Movement(100)	Hygiene (45)	Study/Homework (30)	Travelling (25)
8	Sleep (780)	Physical Activity with less Movement(225)	Physical activity with more Movement(160)	Meals (140)	Hygiene (90)	Travelling (45)	Study/Homework (0)

What Activities are Carried Out with or Without Accompaniment and What are the Accompaniments for the Activities Carried Out During Weekdays and Weekends?

Regarding the activities carried out with accompaniment, it should be pointed out that: subject 1 showed a lack of autonomy in carrying out personal hygiene, in housework and studying, being assisted mainly by his father, not revealing independence of mobility and requiring accompaniment mainly by the family; subject 2 must always be accompanied (by family members and health technicians), despite being able to perform basic activities such as hygiene, meals and sleeping alone, but demonstrating that he or she is completely dependent on the adult for routes and in the various places they frequently visit; subject 3 revealed autonomy in the accomplishment of most of their activities, although it was not possible to prove independence of mobility during the week, analysing their routes these were always by car and in the activities was accompanied by the family and by their tutor; subject 4 shows autonomy in the performance of his/her activities and independence of mobility, but is often accompanied by family and health technicians; subject 5 showed little autonomy since in activities such as personal hygiene, homework and trips to school they need the accompaniment of the home helpers; subject 6 is more autonomous because the only activity that needs accompaniment is the travelling, which is done by the father and the grandparents, although in physical activities with less movement they enjoy the company of their sister, which is justified by the relationship between the two; subject 7 also showed little autonomy since they are always accompanied by their mother in personal hygiene activities and in the trips; Finally, subject 8 is also not very autonomous, since they also need to be accompanied by the school's auxiliary worker for the routes between home and school, and the home auxiliary workers for homework and household chores.

What are the Materials/Objects Used in the Different Activities Carried Out?

The materials/objects used in activities related to Physical Activity with less Movement and Physical Activity with more Movement were the following: subject 1, tablet, ball and tennis equipment; subject 2, teddies, dolls, pencils and pens objects that promote little interaction with their peers; subject 3, mobile phone also with little interaction; subject 4, tablet and computer with reduced interaction with peers; subject 5, computer, cars, dolls, ball and swimming material; subject 6, computer, play-station and football and swimming equipment; 7 subject, video, radio, MP3, puppets and judo and swimming material; subject 8, ball, cars, dolls, TV, computer and swimming equipment.

What Activities Carried Out by the Child/Youth Involve Movement?

Activities that involve more movement focus on activities such as those practicing in clubs/associations such as tennis (subject1), football (subject 6), judo (subject 7) and swimming (subjects 5, 6, 7 and 8) ; therapies such as psychomotricity (subject 2), occupational therapy (subject 2), hippotherapy (subjects 3, 5 and 8) and physiotherapy (subjects 4 and 6); outdoor games (subjects 1, 5, 6 and 8)), outdoor excursions (subject 3) and shopping (subjects 3 and 4); and finally, the travelling on foot in some short journeys (subjects 1, 2, 4 and 6).

What Places are Frequented in Daily Routines?

The places visited were the school, the house (own or the grandparents) and the specific places where they carry out the activities practiced in clubs/associations, therapies, tutoring, catechesis and music conservatory. At **the weekend**, it is at home that they spend most of their time. However, there were other places, such as the garden (subject 5), the park (subject 1 and 5), the shopping centre (subjects 2, 3 and 4), the market (subject 6), recreation (subject 8) and other outdoor places (subject 3).

What are the Most Important/Significant Places?

For subjects 1, 2, 6 and 7, the house was referred to as their preferred site. Subjects 3, 4, 5 and 8 reported that although it is at home that they spend most of their time, strolling and playing in the park or playground appear as significant aspects and to the subjects.

What and how are the Routes Travelled to go to Different Places?

The routes were home/school and vice versa and the specific paths where they carry out the different activities (therapies, activities in clubs/associations, music conservatory, tutoring and catechesis). The routes were carried out mainly by car or by school transport (subjects 5 and 8), in the company of family members or school helpers (subjects 5 and 8). Four of the subjects (1, 2, 4 and 6) also walked on trips to school and to other places where they carry out activities.

What are the Main Obstacles Encountered in the Routes?

For subjects 1, 2, 5 and 8 the characteristics associated with their problems it is the age that constitutes the greatest obstacle in the completion of the routes, autonomously. Traffic and other hazards (assaults, mistreatment) that may occur during journeys are also barriers. Age seems to be a facilitator in the independence of mobility observed in subjects 3, 4, 6 and 7.

CONCLUDING REMARKS

From the objectives outlined for this study, we present the main conclusions:

1 - The activities performed indoors, during the week (weekdays and weekend) were *Physical Activities with less Movement; To sleep; Meals; Teaching/Homework and Hygiene. The Physical Activities with less Movement* carried out focused mainly on watching TV, playing with the tablet and/or computer and/or mobile phone, listening to music, watching videos and playing with objects. Activities carried out **outside the home** were mainly *Physical Activities with more Movement* (such as those practiced outdoors, in clubs/associations and therapies) and *Travelling* such as travelling on foot.

2 - Regarding the time spent on activities, excluding time spent sleeping, the subjects spent more time on *Physical Activities with less Movement* and *Meals,* either on weekdays or on weekends. During the week there is also a time dedicated to *Physical Activities with more Movement* by seven subjects, but at the end of the week, only five subjects perform activities of this nature.

3 - The accompanying persons in the different activities were, above all, family members or auxiliary staff (for those who are institutionalized), therapist technicians and specific accompanying persons, namely teachers (tennis, football, swimming, judo, tutoring, music conservatory) and catechist.

4 - Activities that involve movement are related to those practiced in clubs/associations (football, tennis, swimming and judo), therapies (psycho-motor, hippotherapy, occupational therapy, physiotherapy), outdoor games in the park and yard (playing hide and seek, playing football, playing catch), shopping at the Shopping Centre and walking, especially between school-home-school.

5 - The places frequented in the daily routines **during the weekdays**, were to school, their house and the specific places where they carry out the activities like music conservatory, tutoring, catechesis, activities in clubs/associations and therapies. At the weekend, it is at home that they spend most of their time. The most important/significant place for the children/young people was their home.

6 - The routes made were limited to the home-school-house route and to the specific routes where they carry out the different activities. The specific routes were carried out mainly by car, in the company of relatives or home helpers, and the home-school-house routes were performed by half of the subjects also on foot and two of them without the presence of any adult.

7 - The materials/objects used in the activities were mainly electronic media such as mobile phone, tablet and computer, (which promote little interaction with the parents), dolls, balls, cars to play with their friends and the materials used in the specific activities.

8 - The main obstacles during the routes were related to the characteristics

associated with pathologies, traffic and other hazards.

CONSENT FOR PUBLICATION

Not applicable.

CONFLICT OF INTEREST

The author confirms that this chapter contents have no conflict of interest.

ACKNOWLEDGEMENTS

Declared none.

REFERENCES

Apolo, A. (2010). *Análise da Mobilidade de Pessoas com Deficiência - Estudo de Caso. Dissertação para obtenção do grau de Mestre em Engenharia na Área de Especialização de Vias de Comunicação e Transportes.*. Instituto Superior de Engenharia de Lisboa.

Arez, A., Neto, C. (2000). Independência de mobilidade em crianças de meios urbanos distintos. In: Mendes, R., Barreiros, J., Vasconcelos, O., (Eds.), *Estudos em Desenvolvimento Motor da Criança V* (pp. 174-184). Escola Superior de Educação de Coimbra.

Barbosa-Ducharne, M., Cruz, O., Marinho, S., Grande, S. (2012). Estilos de vida adolescente: exploração de rotinas diárias à semana e ao fim de semana. *Revista Amazônica.* Ano 5, Vol VIII, n.º 1, pág. 149-172.

Barbosa, A. (2016). Mobilidade urbana para pessoas com deficiência no Brasil: um estudo em blogs. *Urbe - Revista Brasileira de Gestão Urbana.* vol. 8, núm. 1, enero-abril, pp. 142-154.

Bogdan, R., Biklen, S. (1994). *Investigação Qualitativa em Educação – Uma Introdução à Teoria e aos Métodos.* Porto: Porto Editora.

Brandão, B., Gonçalves, D., Medeiros, P. (2006). Rotinas na Aprendizagem *Cadernos de Estudo, 4*, 23-29.

Chombart De Lauwe, M. J., Bonnin, P., Mayeur, M., Perrot, M., Soudiere, M. (1976). *Enfant en jeu – les pratiques des enfants durant leur temps libre en fonction des tipes d`environement et des idèologies.* Paris: Centre D`Etologi Sociale et de Psichosociologie, ECNRS.

Craidy, C., Kaercher, G. (2001). *Educação infantil? Pra que te quero?.* Porto Alegre: Artmed.

Cruz, P. (2011). Ambiente urbano: lugar de restrição espacial e descoberta *de novos* espaços. *Saúde e Sociedade, São Paulo, 20*(3), 702-714.
[http://dx.doi.org/10.1590/S0104-12902011000300015]

Folque, M. (2014). *O Aprender a Aprender No Pré-escolar: O Modelo Pedagógico do Movimento da escola Moderno.* Lisboa: Fundação Calouste Gulbenkian.

Freire, M. (2010). *A inclusão através do Desporto Adaptado: O caso português do Basquetebol em Cadeira de Rodas. Dissertação de Mestrado em Exercício e Saúde em Populações Especiais.*. Faculdade de Ciências do Desporto e Educação Fisica da Universidade de Coimbra.

Gomes, R., Paixão, L. (2013). *Análise da Acessibilidade Física e Arquitetónica de Uma Edificação do Campus da Universidade Estadual de Feira de Santana.*. Belo Horizonte: Universidade Estadual Feira de Santana. Congresso Internacional Interdisciplinar em Sociais e Humanidades.

Gomide, A., Galindo, E. (2013). A mobilidade urbana: uma agenda inconclusa ou o retorno daquilo que não foi. *Estud. Av., 27*(79), 27-39.
[http://dx.doi.org/10.1590/S0103-40142013000300003]

Gonçalves, H. (2014). *Manual de Metodologia da Pesquisa Científica.*. São Paulo: Ed. Avercamp. 2ª ed.

Greguol, M., Gobbi, E., Carraro, A. (2013). Formação de Professores para a Educação Especial: uma Discussão Sobre os Modelos Brasileiro c Italiano. *Revista Brasileira de Educação Especial, 19*(3), 307-324.

Greguol, M. (2017). *Atividades físicas e esportivas e pessoas com deficiência. Relatório Nacional de desenvolvimento humano no Brasil.*. PNUD.

Günther, H. (2003). Mobilidade e affordance como cerne dos estudos pessoa-ambiente. *Estud. Psicol., 8*(2), 273-280.
[http://dx.doi.org/10.1590/S1413-294X2003000200009]

Hohmann, M., Weikart, P. (2011). *Educar a criança.*. Lisboa: Fundação Calouste Gulbenkian.

Interdonato, G., Greguol, M. (2011). Qualidade de Vida e Prática Habitual de Atividade Física em Adolescentes Com Deficiência. *Revista Brasileira Crescimento Desenvolvimento Humano, 21*(2), 282-295.

Jaarsma, E., Dekker, R., Koopmans, S., Dijkstra, P., Geertzen, J. (2014). Barriers to and facilitators of sports participation in people with visual impairments. *Adopt. Phys. Act. Quart, 31*(3), 240-264.

Kirchner, C., Gerber, E., Smith, B. (2008). Designed to deter: community barriers to physical activity for people with visual or motorimpairments. *Am. J. Prevent. Med., 34*(4), 349-352.

Lee, M., Zhu, W., Ackley-Holbrook, E., Brower, D., McMurray, B. (2014). Calibration and validation of the Physical Activity Barrier Scale for persons who are blind or visually impaired. *Disabil. Health J., 7*(3), 309-317.
[http://dx.doi.org/10.1016/j.dhjo.2014.02.004]

Lopes, C. (2013). *Rotinas de vida, autonomia e mobilidade de jovens em contexto urbano. Dissertação de Mestrado em Educação para a Saúde.*. Portugal: Instituto Politécnico de Coimbra. Escola Superior de Tecnologia.

Magalhães, M., Aragão, J., Yamashita, Y. (2013). Definições formais de mobilidade e acessibilidade apoiadas na teoria de sistemas de Mário Bunge.Paranoá: *Cadernos de Arquitetura e Urbanismo, (9)*, 1-14.

Mahoney, J., Harris, A., Eccles, J. (2006). Organized activity participation, positive youth development, and the over-scheduling hypothesis. *Social Policy Report: Giving child and youth development knowledge away, , 3-30.

Marconi, M., Lakatos, E. (1996). *Técnicas de pesquisa.*. São Paulo: Atlas. 3ª ed.

Marmeleira, J., Laranjo, L., Marques, O., Pereira, C. (2014). Physical activitypatterns in adults who are blind as assessed by accelerometry. *Adopt. Phys. Activ. Quart., 31*, 283, 293.

Martins, D. (2018). *Rotinas de Vida Diária de Crianças/Jovens com NEE - Estudo de Caso. Dissertação Mestrado em Educação Especial no Domínio Cognitivo e Motor.* Escola Superior de Educação do Instituto Politécnico de Castelo Branco.

Moreno, D. (2009). *Jogo de atividade física e a influência de variáveis biossociais na vida quotidiana de crianças em meio urbano. Tese de Doutoramento em Motricidade Humana na especialidade de Ciências da Motricidade.* Universidade Técnica de Lisboa. Faculdade de Motricidade Humana.

Marmeleira, J., Fernandes, J., Ribeiro, N., Teixeira, J., Filho, P. (2018). Barreiras para a prática de atividade física em pessoas com deficiência visual. *Revista Brasileira de Ciências do Esporte, 40*(2), 197-204.
[http://dx.doi.org/10.1016/j.rbce.2017.12.001]

Pereira, A. (2014). *O contributo das rotinas diárias para o desenvolvimento da autonomia das crianças. Dissertação de Mestrado em Educação Pré-escolar.* Escola Superior de Educação do Instituto Politécnico de Portalegre.

Pinto, M. (1995). *A televisão no quotidiano das crianças. Tese de Doutoramento em Ciências da Comunicação.* Braga: Instituto de Ciências Sociais da Universidade do Minho.

Rimmer, J., Riley, B., Wang, E., Rauworth, A., Jurkowski, J. (2004). Physical activity participation among persons with disabilities: barriers and facilitators. *Am.J. Prevent. Med., 26*(5), 419-425.

Santos, I. (2016). *Rotinas de Vida Diária de Crianças Portadoras de Deficiência - estudo de caso. Dissertação Mestrado em Atividade Física na especialidade em Desporto Adaptado.* Escola Superior de Educação do Instituto Politécnico de Castelo Branco.

Selltiz, C., Jahoda, M., Deutsch, M., Cook, S. (1974). *Métodos de Pesquisa nas Rela-ções Sociais.* E.P.U., S. Paulo. 4ª Ed.

Serrano, J. (2003). *Mudanças sociais e estilos de vida no desenvolvimento da criança. Estudo do nível de independência de mobilidade e da atividade física nas rotinas de vida quotidiana em crianças de 8, 10 e 12 anos de idade no meio urbano. Tese de Doutoramento em Motricidade Humana na especialidade de Ciências da Motricidade.* Universidade Técnica de Lisboa. Faculdade de Motricidade Humana.

Teixeira, O. (2014). *Mobilidade e acessibilidade urbana - Estudo de caso do Município de Viana. Dissertação de Mestrado em Gestão Autárquica..* Escola de Educação, Gestão, Design, Engenharia, Aeronáutica e Design - Instituto Superior de Educação e Ciências.

Teles, P. (2005). *Os Territórios (Sociais) da Mobilidade – Um Desafio para a Área Metropolitana do Porto..* Aveiro: Edições Lugar do Plano.

Triviños, A. (1992). *Introdução à pesquisa em ciências sociais: a pesquisa qualitativa em educação.* São Paulo: Atlas. 3ª ed.

Warburton, D., Nicol, C., Bredin, S. (2006). Health benefits of physical activity: the evidence. *Can. Med. Assoc. J., 174*(6), 801, 809.

WHO. (2011). *International Classification of Functioning, Disability and Health (ICF). World report on disability.* World Health Organization, The World Bank.

Yin, K. (1994). *Case Study Research: Design and Methods.* (2nd ed.). Thousand Oaks: Sage Publications.

CHAPTER 5

Sensory Integration and the Child with Autism Spectrum Disorders

Helena S. Reis[1,*] and **Pedro J. Bargão**[2]

[1] *School of Health Sciences & ciTechCare - Center for Innovative Care and Health Technology, Polytechnic of Leiria, Portugal*

[2] *School of Health Sciences, Polytechnic of Leiria, Portugal*

Abstract: Since the disorder was first identified, difficulty in processing, integrating and responding to sensory stimuli has been described as a feature of autism spectrum disorders (ASD). Current estimates show that between 42 and 98% of children with ASD demonstrate these sensory difficulties and sensory features (*i.e.*: hyper- or hyporeactivity to sensory input or unusual interest in the sensory aspects of the environment) that are now included as one of four possible manifestations of 'Restricted, Repetitive Patterns of Behavior, Interests, or Activities' (American Psychiatric Association, 2013). Families report that behaviours associated with difficulties in processing and integrating sensory information create social isolation for them and their child, restrict participation in daily living activities and impact social engagement. Three types of Sensory Processing disorders are distinguished: (1) sensory modulation disorders, which affect the regulation of the level or intensity of the response that occurs in the presence of the sensory information, thus differentiating between over-responsiveness, under-responsiveness and sensory seeking, (2) sensory discrimination disorders, which affect the ability to distinguish and identify sensory inputs, and (3) sensorimotor integration disorders, which involve a difficulty in transforming sensations into motor responses, including postural disorders with a sensory basis and developmental dyspraxia, in which ideation and motor planning are compromised, producing difficulties in learning new motor tasks. Consequently, interventions to address problems associated with difficulty processing sensory information, such as occupational therapy using sensory integration are among the most often requested services by parents of children with ASD.

Keywords: Autism Spectrum Disorder, Sensory Integration, Sensory Processing Dysfunction.

INTRODUCTION

Sensory Integration was a theory developed by Jean Ayres around the 1960s, and

* **Corresponding author Helena S. Reis:** School of Health Sciences & ciTechCare - Center for Innovative Care and Health Technology, Polytechnic of Leiria, Portugal; E-mail: helena.s.reis@ipleiria.pt

Samuel Honório, Marco Batista, Helena Mesquita & Jaime Ribeiro (Eds.)

it is defined as the neurological process through which the central nervous system receives, registers and organizes sensory input to create an adapted response of the body to the environment. The spatial and temporal aspects of the data received from different sensory modalities are interpreted, associated and unified, and then a response is produced according to the environment's demands - the adaptive response (Ayres, 1979). Ayres (1972) defines adaptive response as an appropriate action in which the individual successfully responds to any environmental stimulus. Adaptive responses require that the individual tries a type and an amount of sensory stimulation that challenges but does not overload the central nervous system, in which case, the production of an adaptive response is boosted.

Sensory integration is mostly based on three basic senses - tactile, vestibular and proprioceptive. The interconnections between these systems start to take shape before birth and continue to develop as the child matures and interacts with the environment. These three senses are not only interconnected between themselves but also to other brain systems, so this is considered a complex interconnection. They are less familiar systems compared with sight and hearing, but they are fundamental to our basic survival (Ayres, 2005). *Proprioception* is the term used to describe sensations that are received from the tendons, muscles and joints. The proprioceptive system carries information about joint position and movement (Herdman, 2007). The *vestibular system* detects position and movement of the head relative to gravity. Together, the vestibular and proprioceptive systems provide information about the body's position in space, about body parts relative to each other, and about the dynamic movement of the body through space. This information is used to support postural control; balance; and the coordinated movement of the eyes, head, neck, and body. Someone who has precise vestibular and proprioceptive perception is likely to move gracefully, keeping his or her balance while moving with skill and precision. When the vestibular or proprioceptive system is impaired, individuals have difficulty developing a good body scheme. They will have poor balance, poor postural control, difficulty in forming well-lateralized sensorimotor functions, and poorly coordinated movements of the body and limbs, both separately and together (Cullen, 2012).

The visual, olfactory, gustatory and auditory sensory systems - also channels through which we obtain information about the environment - are equally responsible for our adaptive responses to the environment in an adequate way (Hilton *et al.*, 2010). Children and adults with Autism Spectrum Disorder (ASD), as well as other individuals with developmental disorders, may present with a dysfunctional sensory system. Sometimes, one or more senses may be more or less reactive to stimuli. Such sensory problems can be the main reason for behavior such as shifting balance, spinning and flapping hands. Although the receptors of the senses are present in the peripheral nervous system (which excludes the brain and the spinal cord), it is believed that the problem is caused by the neurological dysfunction of the central nervous system - brain (Kuhaneck & Watling, 2010). Reports of individuals with High-Functioning Autism Spectrum Disorder (HFASD) mention that some sensory integration techniques, such as pressure and touch, can facilitate attention and awareness, and reduce the state of general excitement (Murray-Slutsky & Paris, 2000). Temple Grandin, in his book "*Thinking in Pictures*", talks about the anguish and relief of some of his sensory experiences (Grandin, 1995).

Sensory processing refers to the way the brain receives, organizes and interprets sensory input. The reception, modulation, integration and organization of the sensory stimulus, including the behavioral responses to said input, are components of sensory processing (Mailloux, & Smith-Roley, 2001).

An optimal processing ability allows someone to give an adaptive response to the demands of the environment and to adequately take up his or her daily occupations. Any activity undertaken by the individual requires the processing of the sensation, or "sensory integration" (Humphry, 2002; Lane, Young, Baker, & Angley, 2010).

ASD represent a wide range of conditions that manifest themselves in a series of deficits, but sensory issues are now part of the diagnostic criteria of Autism Spectrum Disorder in the most recent description of the disorder in the *Diagnostic and Statistical Manual of Mental Disorders* (5th edition), including hyper- or hypo-reactivity to sensory input or unusual interests in sensory aspects of the environment (*e.g.* apparent indifference to pain/temperature, adverse response to specific sounds or textures, excessive smelling or touching of objects, visual fascination with light or movement) (APA, 2013). We know that the symptoms can vary with different categories, including social interaction, perseveration (repetitive and stereotyped movement), somatosensory disorder (movement or balance shifting frequency), atypical development standards, mood changes (hyper-reactivity or absence of responses to stimuli) and attention and security problems (Pfeiffer, Koening, Kinnealey, Sheppard, & Henderson, 2011). With the growing understanding of neuropsychology in ASD, research has been focusing more on the definition of motor performance and on the sensory processing of these children. Behavioral studies have shown that behavior is not only associated with difficulties in social communication and in restricted interests but also in what concerns the sensory experiences of children with ASD, which are different when compared with typically developing peers (Kuhaneck & Watling, 2010). Children with ASD have difficulty in processing the sensory input and adequately responding to the demands of the environment (Hilton *et al.*, 2010).

SENSORY PROCESSING DYSFUNCTIONS IN ASD

Sensory Processing Dysfunctions have been historically referred to as "Sensory Integration Dysfunctions", but in the last years, the name has been undergoing adjustments (with some controversy in the medical community). Sensory Processing Dysfunctions can lead to sensorimotor problems and learning difficulties of these children. These dysfunctions refer to the way the brain receives and processes the sensory information through the body and the environment, and how it produces an appropriate motor and behavioural response (Davies & Gavin, 2007). Jean Ayres, as a pioneer in this area around the 1960s, coined the expression "Sensory Integration Dysfunctions" (currently "Sensory Processing Disorder"). She found that sensory information can be received by people with Sensory Processing Disorder. The difference is in the way the brain registers, interprets and processes the information, as shown in Table **1**.

Sensory processing dysfunctions include a series of neurological disorders that affect the brain's normal functioning, inhibiting the child's development at the communication and social interaction level (Dunn, 1997; Kranowitz, 2005).

Table 1. Symptoms of Sensory Processing Dysfunction (Adapted from Kranowitz, C., 2005).

Sensory Modality	Some Symptoms
Auditory	Responds negatively to unexpected or very loud noises Covers ears with hands Can't work with background noise Seems withdrawn in an active environment
Visual	Prefers to be in the dark Avoids intense light Stares at people or objects Avoids eye contact
Gustatory/olfactory	Avoids specific tastes/smells that are part of children's food Frequently smells objects Craves specific tastes or smells Seems unable to smell strong odors
Proprioceptive	Constantly tries all kinds of movement Frequently runs into people, furniture, objects, even in familiar situations Seems to have weak muscles, is easily tired, has low endurance Walks on tiptoes
Vestibular	Gets nervous when feet no longer touch the ground Avoids jumping/climbing Avoids playground equipment Tries all kinds of movement, and that interferes with daily routines Takes excessive risks when playing, unaware of the danger Walks on tiptoes

(Table 1) cont.....

Sensory Modality	Some Symptoms
Tactile	Avoids touching certain materials (glue, fingerpaint, sand, modeling doughs) Is sensitive to a specific fabric Constantly needs to touch people and objects Avoids walking barefoot, especially on grass or sand Has high tolerance to pain and temperature

According to Schaaf and Nightlinger (2007), there are 3 types of Sensory Processing Dysfunctions:

Type I - *Sensory Modulation Dysfunction* - Over- or Under-responsivity to a sensory stimulus or sensory seeking. This group may include a pattern of fear and/or anxiety behavior and thoughts including negative behavior and/or stubbornness and self-absorption on the part of the child that makes engagement hard. It also includes behavior that makes the child suffer when actively seeking an activity.

Type II - *Sensory-Motor Dysfunction* - It reveals that the child's motor output is disorganized as the result of incorrect processing of the sensory information, affecting the changes at the level of postural control and/or dyspraxia.

Type III - *Sensory Discrimination Dysfunction* - Sensory discrimination or incorrect processing of the sensory information. The incorrect processing of the auditory or visual input can, for instance, translate into distraction, disorganization and poor school performance.

Dysfunctions in sensory and perceptive processing, as well as in communication and neurological functioning, result in several functional behavioral limitations, as is the case of children with ASD (Abelenda, Mailloux, & Roley, 2015; Ben-Sasson *et al.*, 2007).

Sensory Processing Dysfunctions (SPD) are frequently described in these children, and the literature mentions that 42% to 98% of children with ASD present with this type of dysfunction (Baranek, 2002; Case-Smith, Weaver, & Fristad, 2015). Therefore, children with ASD show difficulty in regulating responses to sensations and may use self-stimulation to compensate for the sensory input limited to their neurological threshold or to avoid over-stimulation. This is also seen as a self-regulated strategy. (Bogdashina, 2003; Tomchek & Dunn, 2007).

Self-regulation is a key concept of development contributing to attention, behavior and social skills. *Regulatory processes* are a varied, widespread and diverse set of constructs, including neurophysiological system control and organization, which involve arousal and sensory-motor modulation. There is no comprehensive definition of self-regulation, but it is well accepted that regulatory processes allow an individual to sustain physiological homeostasis, as well as to self-organize in various contexts using cognitive, sensory, motor, attention and emotional strategies (Fieldman, 2009).

Regulatory functions span from physiology to behavior, and sensation plays a major role in enhancing, sustaining and interfering with self-regulation across all dimensions. Common examples include rocking, patting, or swaddling an infant; watching nature scenes on television; smelling roses; and receiving a massage. Sensory regulation deficits are documented in humans and primates (Schneider *et al.*, 2007). Hierarchical-integrative perspectives highlight that emotional, attentional, and self-regulatory functions build on each other as a foundation for higher-level cognitive, social and behavioral regulatory functions. Dysregulated behaviors are common in children with ASD and are regularly seen as irregular sensory responsiveness or unusual sensory seeking behaviors. Atypical sensory regulation affects a child's ability to benefit from sensory co-regulation strategies initiated by caregivers, such as swaddling and rocking for calming. Linked to stress responses, diminished regulatory capacities increase stress, lower immune function and, when they are severe, affect memory and executive functions (Gilotty, Kenworthy, Sirian, Black, & Wagner, 2002).

Sensory Modulation Profiles in ASD

The existing interaction between neuroscience and behavioral concepts helps us interpret the behavior and performance of children. Through neuroscience, one is able to understand how sensory receptors receive and transmit stimuli, how the central nervous system (CNS) decodes and interprets information, and how that same information is used in a motor output (Dunn, 1997). The most recent literature on neuroscience also highlights the importance of the modulation of all sensory information input as a part of CNS' adjusted functioning.

Modulation is the ability to monitor and regulate the sensory information in order to produce an adaptive response to a particular stimulus; it is the regulation between the facilitation and inhibition of the stimulus input (Myles, Cook, Miller, Rinner, & Robbins, 2001). "When an individual over-responds, under-responds or fluctuates in response to the sensory input in a way that is inappropriate for that input, it is said that he or she presents with a modulation disorder" (Koomar, & Bundy, 1991, p. 268).

The key to the neurophysiological process related to modulation is *habituation* and *sensitization*. *Habituation* is considered as the CNS' simplest way to learn, and it occurs when nerve cells and the CNS' systems recognize the stimulus as something familiar, which means the transmission of information to the cells to continue answering the stimulus is reduced (Dunn, 1997) .

Sensitization in the CNS expresses an exaggerated cell response. During sensitization, the CNS recognizes the stimulus as something important or potentially threatening and produces an exaggerated response. Children use this neurophysiological way to stay alert and attentive to what is happening around them.

According to Dunn (1997) when children with ASD have a poor modulation between habituation and sensitization, they present with non-adaptive responses, such as hyperactivity or excitement (*e.g.* over-Sensitization - low neurological threshold), or lethargy or withdrawal (*e.g.* over-Habituation - high neurological threshold), as shown in Table **2**.

Table 2. Sensory Modulation Profiles (Adapted from Williamson, G., & Anzalone, M., 2001, p.33).

Neurological Threshold	Behavioral Response	
	Responds in accordance with his or her neurological threshold	Responds by adjusting his or her neurological threshold
High (Habituation)	Poor Registration	Sensory Seeking
Low (Sensitization)	Sensitive to stimulus	Sensory Avoidance

The sensory processing model by Dunn (1997) refers to the relation between the neurological threshold and self-regulation strategies for the child to obtain an adaptive behavior. The neurological threshold can be high - when the intensity of the stimulation needs to be high for the child to respond - or low - when the intensity of the stimulation needs to be low to elicit a response. The continuity of self-regulation varies between passive strategies (children who do not act against unpleasant stimuli) and active (children who act so as to control the amount and type of sensory input) (Dunn, 1997; Hochhauser & Engel-Yeger, 2010).

Through this interaction, the model by Dunn (2007a) classifies sensory processing patterns in four subtypes:

(1) *Sensory Seeking*, represents a high neurological threshold with active self-regulation strategies. These children engage in actions in an energetic way in order to make the sensations they receive more intense, which means they have a greater tendency to shift attention during learning activities and social interactions;

(2) *Sensory Avoidance* includes a low neurological threshold and active self-

regulation strategies. The behavior of these children is characterized by rigid and inflexible rituals, with difficulty in transitions. They usually feel threatened by the "sensation" and therefore tend to adopt an avoiding behavior toward activities (Dunn, 2007b);

(3) *Sensory Sensitivity* includes low neurological thresholds with passive self-regulation strategies. These children quickly respond to sensations, with a higher intensity and longer duration than children with typical sensory responsiveness. They are children who can offer active, impulsive or aggressive responses, or even withdraw from the environment in order to avoid the sensation (Dunn, 2007b);

(4) *Low Registration* represents a high neurological threshold with passive self-regulation strategies. These children tend to adopt a passive response to the environment by not responding or not giving importance to the environment's sensory stimuli. It seems that they do not detect the input of the sensory information and show a deficit in their responses. Because of this, they appear to be introvert, apathetic or lethargic children with a deficit in the "*inner drive*" to start exploring (Dunn, 2007b).

Research shows that children with ASD present with atypical sensory processing, which can be observed through sensory *under-responsivity* (*e.g.* they seem not to react to pain; they are confused by loud sounds or do not respond when hearing their name), *over-responsivity* to sensory input (*e.g.* aggressive reaction to touch; cover ears against several noises, especially unexpected ones) and/or *sensory-seeking* (*e.g.* engage in self-stimulating activities such as spinning, making sounds, snapping fingers) (Lane, Dennis, & Geraghty, 2011).

SUPPORTING STUDIES

Parents of children with ASD report that the latter present with specific behavior associated with sensory processing dysfunctions such as stereotyped and repetitive behavior and social anxiety (Lane *et al.*, 2011).

These sensory processing dysfunctions in children with ASD are well documented in the literature, be it through direct observation (Baranek, 1999), parent reports (Baranek, David, Poe, Stone, & Watson, 2006), or descriptions of these difficulties by the children themselves (Grandin, 1992, 1995). In fact, sensory processing dysfunctions are described more frequently in the tactile, visual and auditory systems. However, the other systems usually also show processing changes (Kuhaneck, & Watling, 2010). Several researchers report that auditory processing deficits in children with ASD can vary with over-responsive, under-responsive or even fluctuating responses (Kuhaneck, & Watling, 2010). A study carried out by Greenspan and Wieder (1997) of 200 children with ASD reveals that 100% of the participants show difficulties in auditory processing. Another study shows that 134 of 233 parents (57.5%) of children with ASD report that their child is sensitive to sound, with extreme sensitivity to daily environment noise (doorbells, cars, airplanes, motorcycles) (Gillberg *et al.*, 1990).

Auditory hypo-reactivity has also been described in the literature (Baranek, 1999) and a reduction in the response when hearing their name, as well as a decrease in responses, not only to verbal command but also to noises in general, is often found in these children. This hypo-reactivity should be taken into consideration when making an early diagnosis, seeing that most of these children seem to present with apparent deafness before being diagnosed with ASD (Wing, 1966).

Regarding the visual system, research has produced paradoxical responses. The avoidance of eye contact and the inefficient use of sight have been described as the difficulties found in these children, often classified under the social difficulty category. However, many authors explain the eye contact reduction as a self-regulation mechanism that compensates for the visual input modulation problems. Consequently, this difficulty is better categorized in the context of sensory dysfunctions (Gillberg, & Coleman, 2000; Gillberg *et al.*, 1990). Furthermore, one can also find studies revealing that these children make unusual eye contact with objects (*e.g.* looking at objects out of the corner of their eye, moving fingers in front of their eyes, turning objects) (Lord, Rutter, & Couteur, 1994).

Tactile hypersensitivity is also common in children with ASD (Baranek, Foster, & Berkson, 1997; Cesaroni, & Garber, 1991; Grandin, 1992, 1995) and it has been associated with stereotyped behaviour (Baranek *et al.*, 1997). In this study, children with ASD and tactile defensiveness revealed a greater rigidity and inflexibility of behavior, repetitive verbalizations, visual stereotypies and poor affective ability, and these kinds of behavior are most of the time associated with early ASD diagnosis.

Delacato (1974) was one of the first researchers to suggest that the hyper- and hyposensitivity experienced by children with ASD caused the withdrawal of social interaction and in stereotyped behavior and communication (or self-stimulation). Self-stimulating behavior has been described by this author as a defense mechanism of hyper- or hyposensitivity, highlighting that very often, children engage in this behavior (*i.e.* spinning, shifting balance, flapping hands, drumming fingers, watching objects spin) as an involuntary strategy, in order to deal with the "unwanted sensory stimulation" (hypersensitivity) or lack of it (hyposensitivity). This means that it does not matter how "irritating" or "insignificant" these kinds of behavior may seem, and that it is fruitless to try to suppress them without understanding why they are happening and introducing experiences with the same function (Bogdashina, 2003).

Praxis is also typically difficult for children with ASD. Praxis is the ability to have an idea and plan about a future novel activity that involves deciding what to do and how to do it. Although routine and stereotyped motor activities that do not require praxis, such as walking, running and climbing, are typically easy for individuals with ASD, motor activities that require adaptation, such as building models or using tools, appear to be difficult (Abelenda *et al.*, 2015; Schaaf *et al.*, 2013; Schaaf & Nightlinger, 2007). Motor execution is frequently intact, suggesting that once children with ASD learn a motor skill, their actions can look exquisitely smooth and coordinated. However, specific aspects of praxis, such as timing, sequencing, initiating and transitioning are commonly difficult for these children (Abelenda *et al.*, 2015).

Several studies have demonstrated poor imitative abilities in individuals with ASD (Baranek, 1999, 2002). A disorder in the drive to engage, coupled with poor imitation and deficits in sensory processing, creates a high likelihood of poor praxis abilities (Ayres, 1972). Parahm *et al.* (2011) reported that praxis scores were constantly and significantly lower in children with ASD compared with a matched sample of typically developing children. A study identified similar findings showing significant deficits in sensory-perceptual skills, as well as motor and praxis skills, in children with ASD (Mailloux *et al.*, 2011). In particular, the Oral Praxis Test (Ayres, 1989), a test of the ability to imitate mouth, lip and tongue movements, significantly discriminated between typical children and those with ASD. This finding is consistent with others that have found deficits in the ability to make and imitate facial gestures (Ozonoff, Young, Rogers, & Rozga, 2011)

To optimize the inclusion of these children in society, one should examine how the processing abilities affect their patterns of participation in everyday life. This fact coincides with the concept of the World Health Organization (WHO, 2001), which emphasizes the importance of mentioning the relationship between performance difficulties and participation in activities of daily living (ALDs). It is in participation, defined by the WHO as a vital part of human development and life experiences in which abilities and skills are acquired, that significant life goals are identified.

Existing studies show that children with developmental delays have a lower participation in activities of daily living compared with children with typical development (Ashburner, Ziviani, & Rodger, 2008), and that children with ASD, in particular, participate in an even more restricted way in leisure activities when compared with their peers who suffer from other disorders.

Sensitivity to taste and smell has been associated with a reduced level of participation in the activities of children with high-functioning ASD, especially in activities that imply strong odours (*e.g.* meals, activities with animals). This same study also showed that children with ASD and vestibular (movement) hypersensitivity prefer to participate more in sedentary activities at home, such as watching TV, playing computer games and problem-solving games. In other words, activities that do not involve movement and which are carried out in a more protected, safer and controlled environment, reduce the child's exposure to "unpleasant" sensory stimuli, including movement (Ashburner *et al.*, 2008; Kuhaneck, & Watling, 2010).

When a child is diagnosed with ASD, interventions usually focus on the development of educational and behavioral abilities as a priority in order to develop the child's communication and interaction skills, sometimes without considering his or her sensory specificities and needs (Bogdashina, 2003).

Although sensory processing dysfunctions are not yet an integral part of standardized diagnostic manuals, such as DSM 5 and ICD 10, this designation has been used by many clinicians who refer to children who have difficulty processing and responding to sensory information inputs from the environment. Whereas some researchers defend that sensory processing dysfunctions are a different diagnosis, others consider that the differences observed in sensory responsivity are characteristic of other diagnoses (Keane, 2009). The American Academy of Pediatrics, for instance, is against the exclusive diagnosis of the Sensory Processing Dysfunctions, unless they are considered symptoms of ASD, Attention Deficit and Hyperactivity, Motor Coordination Disorder or Anxiety Disorder in the child. The American Psychiatric Association has also recently rejected the inclusion of Sensory Processing Dysfunctions in the new DSM-5, saying that there are still not many studies recognizing this category as a separate diagnosis (Keane, 2009).

Although there is still some resistance from certain authors and entities to recognize these dysfunctions, authors such as Stanley Greenspan include sensory processing dysfunctions in the Diagnostic Manual for Infancy and Early Childhood (Zero To Three, 1994) and still consider sensory processing dysfunctions as Regulation Disorders of Sensory Processing in the Zero to Three Diagnostic Classification (N. Guédeney *et al.*, 2003).

The issue of the diagnostic classification of infant mental disorders is the object of controversy and debate (Gonçalves, & Caldeira da Silva, 2003). Proving it is, on one hand, the diversity of classification systems (Mazet, 1998), which one might call "private" (Hersov, Rutter, & Taylor, 1994) due to their close connection to the psychopathological theoretical framework of their authors, whose general application is difficult (Gonçalves, & Caldeira da Silva, 2003). On the other hand, this is visible in difficulty defining the "diagnostic application object" and reaching some consensus to try to solve the conflict between psychopathology and diagnostic classification (A. Guédeney, 1998).

In fact, many professionals have been showing some lack of interest and even resistance to the application of diagnostic classification systems in infant mental health. The Zero to Three Diagnostic Classification (1994, 2005) has therefore gained special attention and is used by teams that are involved, for the most part, in psychoanalytical training and a psychodynamically oriented practice. They have confirmed the importance of relationship disorders in triggering psychopathological disorders in infants, in the mostly preventive quality of interventions, and in the fact that the intervention's orientation depends a lot more on the mental functioning of an infant, within the scope of its relationship with the parents, than on the symptomatic or behavioral manifestations it may present with (Gonçalves, & Caldeira da Silva, 2003).

EVALUATION

During an occupational therapy evaluation, it is essential to determine the desired activities or occupations of the child and family, and the ways in which occupational therapy can benefit their health and participation in daily life activities. An occupation-centered evaluation considers the effect that engaging in daily activities has on the well-being of these individuals and on the environment of contexts that surround them. Evaluating children with ASD presents many challenges. For children with ASD who are able to reliably respond in a standardized test situation, the Sensory Integration and Praxis Test (Ayres, 1989) offers the most comprehensive measures of sensory integration functions. More frequently, however, children with ASD have difficulties with cognition, language learning, attention, transitions, and social reciprocity that rule out the use of standardized tests. In this case, the therapist relies on observations of those elements of sensory integration and praxis without the benefit of normative comparisons. Many aspects of sensory integration functions can be assessed through structured and unstructured observations of the child. The parent's and caregiver's narratives are an essential part of the assessment of children with ASD. During interviews, significant individuals in the child's life are asked to describe what the child can and cannot do in everyday life and to describe the context in which the child is performing. Structured observations are conducted in both typical and clinical settings by the therapist. The STEP-SI (sensations, task, environment, predictability, self-monitoring and interactions) clinical reasoning model has been proposed as a method to structure ongoing observation and decision making (Miller, Willbarger, Stachouse, & Trunnel, 2001). Whether standardized or non-standardized assessments are feasible for the child, the following types of information will be helpful in attaining a more complete understanding of children with ASD:

1) Does the child show patterns of under- or over-responsivity to certain types of sensory experiences? What behaviors generally signal that the child is reacting appropriately or inappropriately to sensory experiences? What types of reactions do the child tend to show in relation to which conditions (*e.g.* sleep-wake cycles, hunger, illness, time of day, environmental setting)?

2) Does the child have functional perception and discrimination of specific information from various sensory systems? Do test scores or functional performance indicates signs of poor discriminative ability?

3) What does the child do in unfamiliar or novel environments? Does the child show curiosity and exploratory play? Does the child demonstrate ideation about how to use novel toys or objects? Is the child generally purposeful in activities? Does the child show self-initiation play?

4) Does the child demonstrate adequate skills for play and work? How does the child use utensils and materials? Do any strength or muscle tone issues interfere with performance? Is the child able to coordinate both sides of the body in activities such as cutting, writing, pedaling and swimming?

5) Can the child imitate actions? Does the child follow directions that are given verbally? Can the child complete sequences of actions?

6) How does the child relate to other people in an environment? Does the child appear to regard others? Does the child show interest in watching peers? Does the child show interest in interacting with peers? Does the child initiate interaction with others?

7) How does the environment help or hinder the child's level of comfort, organization, attention and learning? Are the child's caregivers informed about the child's abilities, level of responsivity and areas of challenge? What compensatory strategies and environmental accommodations are available for the child?

INTERVENTION

Occupational therapy programs are tailormade for the specific child and his or her family based on the individual's occupational performance. Because disorders of sensory integration and praxis are prevalent among individuals with ASD, it is difficult to imagine a comprehensive therapy program that would not include at least some components of the sensory integration framework. Ayres Sensory Integration uses a variety of strategies to address the range of disorders in sensory integration and praxis that are common in individuals with ASD. When using the Ayres Sensory Integration frame of reference alone or in combination with other methods of occupational therapy intervention, the overarching goal of an occupational therapist is to establish or restore a healthy lifestyle for the child and child's family by engaging the child in meaningful occupations (Case-Smith *et al.*, 2015; Reis, Pereira, & Almeida, 2018).

Ayres (1972) declared the use of this intervention to be both an art and a science. The artistry emerges with the therapist and the child creating a new scenario each time they engage in therapeutic activities within the context of the play. This scenario unfolds as a consequence of the existing state of the child, his or her ability to handle novelty and challenge that day, and the skilfulness of the therapist to guide and support the child's emerging competencies (Ayres, 1972; Schaaf *et al.*, 2013).

Key constructs guide the therapist in the delivery of therapeutic interactions when using Ayres Sensory Integration. Experts in sensory integration and occupational therapy developed a reliable and valid fidelity measure for use in effectiveness research on Ayres Sensory Integration intervention that outlines essential structural and process elements of the intervention. According to the fidelity measure for Ayres Sensory Integration intervention, these structural elements include:

1) Therapists Qualifications: Occupational therapists, physical therapists and speech and language pathologists can be certified in sensory integration, including the Sensory Integration and Praxis Test (Ayres, 1989) with possibilities for mentorship in this specialized area of practice. The Sensory Integration Certification Program sponsored by the University of Southern California, Division of Occupational Therapy and Western Psychological Services provides training in sensory integration theory and practice, including administering and interpreting the Sensory Integration and Praxis Tests (Ayres, 1989).

2) Review of Client's Records: The therapist must review historical, medical and educational records, assessment data, and relevant professional reports.

3) Of the Physical Environment(s): The physical environment must include adequate space to allow for various types of physical activity; flexible and accessible arrangement of materials; adjustable suspended equipment; and quiet spaces. Equipment requirements include safety features such as mats or crash areas and sensory features such as swinging, bouncing, jumping, climbing and throwing, as well as vibrating toys, visual targets, props to support play, and tools to support daily living skills.

The process elements focus on the therapist's knowledge and skills used in interactions with a child. To facilitate adaptive responses within the meaningful activities with the child, the therapist provides specific sensory opportunities using the following characteristic hallmarks of the sensory integration frame of reference:

• Providing a structured sensory environment that highlights the proprioceptive, vestibular and tactile systems;

• Presenting a range of sensory opportunities (specifically tactile, proprioceptive, and vestibular;

• Using activity and arranging the environment to help the child maintain self-regulation and alertness;

• Challenging postural, ocular, oral, or bilateral motor control;

• Challenging praxis and organization of behavior,

• Ensuring physical safety for the child;

• Arranging the room to engage the child;

• Collaborating on activity choice;

• Creating a context of play;

• Maximizing the child's success;

• Guiding self-organization;

• Fostering therapeutic alliance;

• Supporting optimal arousal by facilitating an adaptive response

• Providing the "just right" challenge

EARLY INTERVENTION IN ASD: WHAT EVIDENCES?

The *National Research Council* (Stansberry-Brunahan & Collet-Klingenberg, 2010) presents six recommendations for the success of the Early Intervention (EI) programs in children with ASD:

1. The intervention should begin as soon as possible from the moment the child is suspected to have ASD;

2. The intervention should include the active engagement of the child with ASD in all the sessions, always considering the child's developmental level and age so that, through meaningful activities, the professionals can reach the planned goals;

3. All interventions should focus on the individual goals of the child with ASD, which have been outlined together with the family;

4. The intervention should involve the family, including the development of its ability to deal with the child with ASD;

5. The intervention should include systematic assessments of the program developed by the professionals and the family so that the development of the child with ASD is evaluated regularly, and for the program to be redefined whenever necessary;

6. The interventions should include opportunities that are inclusive, and the development of the child with ASD should be strengthened, preferably in the child's natural contexts, through the natural interactions with the other children with typical development (nursery, kindergarten, school).

Any EI program in ASD should be built on the family-centered approach, assuming that each family has its skills, which stem from its abilities, talents, resources, values and expectations. This means that the final decision regarding the child or the family is exclusively up to the latter. The role of the professional in the decision-making process should be that of a facilitator of the family's active participation in the promotion of its decision(s) (Dunst, 2000). In this area, one should acknowledge that the decisions made by the family can vary from opportunity to opportunity and that they may depend not only on the family's perception of its resources, concerns and priorities but also on the perceptions of those around it. One of the responsibilities of the professional is to facilitate the availability of means through which those skills can be acknowledged and used (Dunst & Bruder, 2006).

The EI programs have been being proposed as significant programs to reduce the future difficulties of children with ASD. The EI best practice guidelines say that the intervention should begin as soon as possible once the diagnosis is known (ideally 2-4 years of age), that it should use interdisciplinary assessments and custom-made programs, and that these should be used in every context (kindergarten, home, institution/clinic) (Paynter, Scott, Beamish, Duhig, & Heussler, 2012).

The intervention models for ASD vary substantially in terms of the theoretical guidance they are based on, the intervention focus, the intensity, the context in which they are being carried out and in terms of the evidence of the effectiveness of the programs that were drawn up. Several authors (Hemmeter, Joseph, Smith, & Sandall, 2001; McWilliam, Winton, & Crais, 2003) defend the existence of a set of practices that should be the backbone of the whole process of assistance to children with ASD,which include:

- Specialized teams should include professionals from different areas (kindergarten teacher, psychologist, speech therapist and occupational therapist), and they should also include family members to make decisions and work together;

- All team members (including the family) should actively participate in the Early Intervention Individual Plan (EIIP);

- The intervention focuses on the functionality, *i.e.* team members should focus on the child's functioning (*e.g.* engagement, independence, social relations) in his or her natural contexts;

- The team should use a transdisciplinary model to plan and develop the interventions;

- The priorities of the child and family should always be considered as goals to be achieved by the team, whenever they are related to the child's participation in ADLs;

- The routines of the child and the family should be considered as natural intervention opportunities on the part of the team;

- The professionals should enable the families and make them jointly responsible so that they support the development of their children with maximum parental competence, make choices and take decisions without feeling dependent on the professionals;

- The collaboration between the family and the professionals should be effective and constant so that the intended goals and outcomes can be achieved;

- The intervention practices should be individualized and sensitive to the priorities and diversity of each family.

Family-centered practices are recommended by research and have an impact on different areas of the lives of families, namely on the level of their joint accountability, quality of life and of the development of the child (Crais, Roy, &

Free, 2006; Dunst, Trivette, & Hamby, 2007; Pereira, 2009; Warfield, Hauser-Cram, Krauss, Shonkoff, & Upshur, 2004). In the case of children at early ages, in particular, parents can provide extremely valid information about the functioning of their child with ASD in the context of home and the community, which would be extremely hard, if not impossible, to obtain by another team member.

One of the great difficulties among children with ASD is the generalization of the abilities that have been acquired. Therefore, skills that have been demonstrated in specific contexts are not, most of the times, observed in others. That is why families become the "team members" that can best describe the abilities, challenges and developmental history of their child (Boyd, Odom, Humphreys, & Sam, 2010). The family, by sharing its clear understanding, interests and abilities of its child with ASD, can help professionals in the decision-making process about the most appropriate type of assessment and about the intervention plan to be developed, supporting and collaborating in the full assessment process - child intervention.

The family, as the team member that is closest to the child, is also the most likely to obtain better levels of interaction with the child with ASD and to reach his or her best functioning level (Bagnato, 2008).

CONCLUSION

The recognition of the relevance of the sensory integration framework for children with ASD continues to expand both within the field of occupational therapy and beyond its borders. Sensory integration theory as well as the evaluation and intervention strategies that emanate from this approach provides a unique avenue for enhancing the understanding of, and therefore compassionate intervention for individuals suffering from this condition. Autism is a lifelong condition for which no intervention approach currently offers a cure. However, the sensory integration framework does provide supportive, pertinent guidance and the hope of improved quality of life for those with ASD as well as for the families and significant others who care for them.

CONSENT FOR PUBLICATION

Not applicable.

CONFLICT OF INTEREST

The author confirms that this chapter contents have no conflict of interest.

ACKNOWLEDGEMENTS

Declared none.

REFERENCES

Abelenda, J., Mailloux, Z., Roley, S. (2015). Dyspraxia in autism spectrum disorders: Evidence and implications. *Spec. Int. Sect. Quart., 38*(3), 1-4.

APA (Ed.). (2013). *Diagnostic and Statistical Manual of Mental Disorders (DSM-5™)* Washington: American Psychiatric Association.

Ayres, J. (1972). *Sensory Integration and Learning Disorders.* Los Angeles: Western Psychological Services.

Ayres, J. (1979). *Sensory Integration and the Child.* Los Angeles: Western Psychological Services.

Ayres, J. (1989). *Sensory Integration and Praxis Test.* Los Angeles: Western Psychological Services.

Ayres, J. (2005). *Sensory Integration and the Child.* Los Angeles, CA: WPS.

Bagnato, S. (2008). *Authentic Assessment for Early Childhood Intervention: Best Practices.* New York: Guilford Press.

Baranek, G.T. (1999). Autism during infancy: a retrospective video analysis of sensory-motor and social behaviors at 9-12 months of age. *J. Autism Dev. Disord., 29*(3), 213-224.
[http://dx.doi.org/10.1023/A:1023080005650] [PMID: 10425584]

Baranek, G.T. (2002). Efficacy of sensory and motor interventions for children with autism. *J. Autism Dev. Disord., 32*(5), 397-422.
[http://dx.doi.org/10.1023/A:1020541906063] [PMID: 12463517]

Ben-Sasson, A., Cermak, S.A., Orsmond, G.I., Tager-Flusberg, H., Carter, A.S., Kadlec, M.B., Dunn, W. (2007). Extreme sensory modulation behaviors in toddlers with autism spectrum disorders. *Am. J. Occup. Ther., 61*(5), 584-592.
[http://dx.doi.org/10.5014/ajot.61.5.584] [PMID: 17944296]

Bogdashina, O. (2003). *Sensory Perceptual Issues in Autism and Asperger Syndrome: Different Sensory Experiences, Different Perceptual Worlds..* London: Jessica Kingsley Publishers.

Boyd, B., Odom, S., Humphreys, B., Sam, A. (2010). Infants and toddlers with autism spectrum disorder: Early identification and early intervention. *J. Early Interv., 32*(2), 75.
[http://dx.doi.org/10.1177/1053815110362690]

Case-Smith, J., Weaver, L.L., Fristad, M.A. (2015). A systematic review of sensory processing interventions for children with autism spectrum disorders. *Autism, 19*(2), 133-148.
[http://dx.doi.org/10.1177/1362361313517762] [PMID: 24477447]

Crais, E.R., Roy, V.P., Free, K. (2006). Parents' and professionals' perceptions of the implementation of family-centered practices in child assessments. *Am. J. Speech Lang. Pathol., 15*(4), 365-377.
[http://dx.doi.org/10.1044/1058-0360(2006/034)] [PMID: 17102147]

Cullen, K.E. (2012). The vestibular system: multimodal integration and encoding of self-motion for motor control. *Trends Neurosci., 35*(3), 185-196.
[http://dx.doi.org/10.1016/j.tins.2011.12.001] [PMID: 22245372]

Davies, P.L., Gavin, W.J. (2007). Validating the diagnosis of sensory processing disorders using EEG technology. *Am. J. Occup. Ther., 61*(2), 176-189.
[http://dx.doi.org/10.5014/ajot.61.2.176] [PMID: 17436840]

Dunn, W. (1997). The impact of sensory processing abilities on the daily lives of young children and their families: A conceptual model. *Infants Young Child., 9*, 23-35.
[http://dx.doi.org/10.1097/00001163-199704000-00005]

Dunn, W. (2007). Supporting children to participate successfully in everyday life by using sensory processing knowledge. *Infants Young Child., 20*(2), 84-101. a
[http://dx.doi.org/10.1097/01.IYC.0000264477.05076.5d]

Dunst, C. (2000). Revisiting "Rethinking Early Intervention". *Top. Early Child. Spec. Educ., 20*(2), 95-104.
[http://dx.doi.org/10.1177/027112140002000205]

Dunst, C., Bruder, M. (2006). Advancing the agenda of service coordination. *J. Early Interv., 28*(3), 175-177.
[http://dx.doi.org/10.1177/105381510602800305]

Dunst, C.J., Trivette, C.M., Hamby, D.W. (2007). Meta-analysis of family-centered helpgiving practices research. *Ment. Retard. Dev. Disabil. Res. Rev., 13*(4), 370-378.
[http://dx.doi.org/10.1002/mrdd.20176] [PMID: 17979208]

Fieldman. (2009). The development of regulatory functions from birth to 5 years: Insights from premature infants. *Child Develop., 80*(2), 544-561.

Gilotty, L., Kenworthy, L., Sirian, L., Black, D.O., Wagner, A.E. (2002). Adaptive skills and executive function in autism spectrum disorders. *Child Neuropsychol., 8*(4), 241-248.
[http://dx.doi.org/10.1076/chin.8.4.241.13504] [PMID: 12759821]

Grandin, T. (1995). *Thinking in pictures.* New York: Bantam Doubleday Dell.

Hemmeter, M., Joseph, G., Smith, B., Sandall, S. (2001). *DEC Recommended Practices Program Assessment: Improving Practices for Young Children with Special Needs and Their Families.* Missoula: Division for Early Childhood.

Herdman, S.J, Blatt, P.J, Schubert, M.C (2000). Vestibular rehabilitation of patients with vestibular hypofunction or with benign paroxysmal positional vertigo. *Curr. Opin. Neurol., 13*(1), 39-43.

Hilton, C.L., Harper, J.D., Kueker, R.H., Lang, A.R., Abbacchi, A.M., Todorov, A., LaVesser, P.D. (2010). Sensory responsiveness as a predictor of social severity in children with high functioning autism spectrum disorders. *J. Autism Dev. Disord., 40*(8), 937-945.
[http://dx.doi.org/10.1007/s10803-010-0944-8] [PMID: 20108030]

Hochhauser, M., Engel-Yeger, B. (2010). Sensory processing abilities and their relation to participation in leisure activities among children with high-functioning autism spectrum disorder (HFASD). *Res. Autism Spectr. Disord., 4*(4), 746-754.
[http://dx.doi.org/10.1016/j.rasd.2010.01.015]

Koomar, J., Bundy, A. (1991). The art of science of creating direct intervention from theory.*Sensory Integration Theory and Practice..* Philadelphia, PA: FA Davis Company..

Kranowitz, C. (2005). *The Out-of-sync Child: Recognizing and Coping With Sensory Integration Dysfunction.* New York: Perigee Books.

Kuhaneck, H.M., Watling, R. (2010). *Autism: a Comprehensive Occupational Therapy Approach.* Bethesda: AOTA PRESS.

Lane, A.E., Dennis, S.J., Geraghty, M.E. (2011). Brief report: Further evidence of sensory subtypes in autism. *J. Autism Dev. Disord., 41*(6), 826-831.
[http://dx.doi.org/10.1007/s10803-010-1103-y] [PMID: 20839041]

Mailloux, Z., Mulligan, S., Roley, S.S., Blanche, E., Cermak, S., Coleman, G.G., Bodison, S., Lane, C.J. (2011). Verification and clarification of patterns of sensory integrative dysfunction. *Am. J. Occup. Ther., 65*(2), 143-151.
[http://dx.doi.org/10.5014/ajot.2011.000752] [PMID: 21476361]

McWilliam, P.J., Winton, P.J., Crais, E.R. (2003). *Estratégias Práticas Para a Intervenção Centrada na Família.* (Vol. 15). Porto: Porto Editora.

Miller, L., Willbarger, J., Stachouse, T., Trunnel, S. (2001). Use of clinical reasoning in occupational therapy:

The STEP-SI Model of sensory modulation dysfunction In Bundy, S., Lane, E. & Murray, E. (Eds.) *Sensory Integration : Theory and Practice.* Philadelphia: F. A. Davis.

Murray-Slutsky, C., Paris, B, (2000), *Exploring the Spectrum of Autism and Pervasive Developmental Disorders: Intervention Strategies.* USA: Therapy Skill Builders.

Myles, B., Cook, K., Miller, N., Rinner, L., Robbins, L. (2001). *Asperger Syndrome and Sensory Issues: Practical Solutions for Making Sense of the World.* Shawnee Mission, Kansas: Autism Asperger Publishing Co..

Young, G.S., Rogers, S.J., Hutman, T., Rozga, A., Sigman, M., Ozonoff, S. (2011). Imitation from 12 to 24 months in autism and typical development: a longitudinal Rasch analysis. *Dev. Psychol., 47*(6), 1565-1578. [http://dx.doi.org/10.1037/a0025418] [PMID: 21910524]

Parham, L.D., Roley, S.S., May-Benson, T.A., Koomar, J., Brett-Green, B., Burke, J.P., Cohn, E.S., Mailloux, Z., Miller, L.J., Schaaf, R.C. (2011). Development of a fidelity measure for research on the effectiveness of the Ayres Sensory Integration intervention. *Am. J. Occup. Ther., 65*(2), 133-142. [http://dx.doi.org/10.5014/ajot.2011.000745] [PMID: 21476360]

Paynter, J., Scott, J., Beamish, W., Duhig, M., Heussler, H. (2012). A pilot study of the effects of an australian centre-based early intervention program for children with autism. *Open Pediatr. Med. J., 6*, 7-14. [http://dx.doi.org/10.2174/1874309901206010007]

Pereira, A. P. (2009). *Práticas Centradas na Família em Intervenção Precoce: Um Estudo Nacional Sobre Práticas Profissionais.* (Tese de Doutoramento), Universidade do Minho.

Pfeiffer, B.A., Koenig, K., Kinnealey, M., Sheppard, M., Henderson, L. (2011). Effectiveness of sensory integration interventions in children with autism spectrum disorders: a pilot study. *Am. J. Occup. Ther., 65*(1), 76-85.
[http://dx.doi.org/10.5014/ajot.2011.09205] [PMID: 21309374]

Reis, H., Pereira, A. P., Almeida, L. (2018). Intervention effects on communication skills and sensory regulation on children with ASD. *J. Occup. Ther. Schools Early Interv.,* 1-14. [http://dx.doi.org/10.1080/19411243.2018.1455552]

Schaaf, R., Benevides, T., Mailloux, Z., Faller, P., Hunt, J., Hooydonk, E.v. (2013). An intervention for sensory difficulties in children with autism: A randomized trial. *J. Autism Dev. Disord., 44*(7), 1493-1506. [http://dx.doi.org/10.1007/s10803-013-1983-8]

Schaaf, R.C., Nightlinger, K.M. (2007). Occupational therapy using a sensory integrative approach: a case study of effectiveness. *Am. J. Occup. Ther., 61*(2), 239-246. [http://dx.doi.org/10.5014/ajot.61.2.239] [PMID: 17436846]

Schneider, M.L., Moore, C.F., Gajewski, L.L., Larson, J.A., Roberts, A.D., Converse, A.K., DeJesus, O.T. (2008). Sensory processing disorder in a primate model: evidence from a longitudinal study of prenatal alcohol and prenatal stress effects. *Child Dev., 79*(1), 100-113. [http://dx.doi.org/10.1111/j.1467-8624.2007.01113.x] [PMID: 18269511]

Stansberry-Brunahan, L.L., Collet-Klingenberg, L.L. (2010). Evidence-based practices for young children with autism spectrum disorders: guidelines and recommendations from the national resource council and national professional development center on autism spectrum disorders. *Int. J. Early Childhood Spec. Educ., 2*, 45-56.

Tomchek, S.D., Dunn, W. (2007). Sensory processing in children with and without autism: a comparative study using the short sensory profile. *Am. J. Occup. Ther., 61*(2), 190-200. [http://dx.doi.org/10.5014/ajot.61.2.190] [PMID: 17436841]

Warfield, M.E., Hauser-Cram, P., Krauss, M.W., Shonkoff, J.P., Upshur, C.C. (2004). The effect of early intervention services on maternal well-being. *Early Intervention: The Essencial Readings.* (pp. 285-308). Malden: Blackwell Publishing. [http://dx.doi.org/10.1002/9780470755778.ch11]

Williamson, G., Anzalone, M. (2001). *Sensory Integration and Self-Regulation in Infants and Toddlers: Helping Very Young Children Interact with Their Environment.*. Washington, DC: ZERO TO THREE.

CHAPTER 6

Combined Interventions on Diabetes

Mônica Braúna[1], Andreia Inácio[1], Catarina Lobão[2], Vânia Ribeiro[1], Ana Lopes[1], Samuel Honório[2] and Jaime Ribeiro[1,3,*]

[1] *School of Health Sciences & ciTechCare - Center for Innovative Care and Health Technology, Polytechnic of Leiria, Portugal*

[2] *Nursing School of Coimbra, UICISA:E - Health Sciences Research Unit: Nursing, Coimbra, Portugal*

[3] *SHERU - Sports, Health and Exercise Research Unit, Polytechnic Institute of Castelo Branco, Portugal*

[4] *CIDTFF - Research Centre on Didactics and Technology in the Education of Trainers -- University of Aveiro, Portugal*

Abstract: Eating habits and modern society have made diabetes a global concern and those who suffer from it are a vulnerable population due to adverse health consequences and functioning limitations. However, prevention and disease management help maintaining quality of life. This chapter brings together professionals from different scientific fields who have embarked on extensive bibliographical research, merging scientific evidence with professional experience. It is possible to verify that the interprofessional work benefits the patient with diabetes, articulating nursing care, nutritional education, practise of adjusted physical activity and the adaptation of environments, occupations and activities supervised by an Occupational Therapist. It is intended that the reader seizes the knowledge of different professionals, use it to their own advantage and help those who need it.

Keywords: Cognitive decline, Diabetes, Dementia, Dietetics and Nutrition, Nursing, Occupational Therapy, Physical exercise, Self-management.

INTRODUCTION

Having diabetes is an increased risk of vulnerability. It is a disease that is often silent and, if not effectively controlled, has serious repercussions on the health condition and quality of life of a person. It is not uncommon to see sequelae in vision and movement (retinopathy and neuropathy) that can cause functional limitations and impair independence and autonomy. It is necessary to intervene in

---

* **Corresponding author Jaime Ribeiro:** School of Health Sciences, Polytechnic of Leiria, Leiria, Portugal; E-mail: jaime.ribeiro@ipleiria.pt

Samuel Honório, Marco Batista, Helena Mesquita & Jaime Ribeiro (Eds.)

primary care for its prevention and minimization of sequelae and, when in more severe cases, intervene to rehabilitate the person, minimize functional issues and prolong quality life.

Diabetes mellitus, seen as a chronic disease, represents a serious and growing public health problem, with numerous complications, both individual and in the community. Its incidence and prevalence are increasing considerably and have reached epidemic proportions. Uncontrolled diabetes can result in devastating complications in various organs and systems of the body including Feet, Kidneys and Eyes (microvascular complications), as well as cause macrovascular complications, which can lead to acute myocardial infarction and stroke. Prevention by changing eating habits and exercise, timely treatment of diabetes complications, and self-management of diabetes tend to provide everyone with a better quality of life as well as better control of the disease.

This chapter aims to show an intervention combined with the vision of the scientific areas of Nursing, Dietetics, Sports and wellness and Occupational Therapy. In this way, in a multidisciplinary approach that combines Occupational Therapy and Physical Education professionals, it is important to list a set of scientific evidence that describes the benefits of exercise and physical activity in minimizing cognitive deterioration due to ageing. It also aims to submit a proposal for an exercise and physical activity program that helps seniors and their formal and informal caregivers.

HEALTH CARE IN DIABETES

Diabetes Mellitus (DM) is a disease known to man since ancient times. It is assumed to be a public health problem and is considered as one of the "epidemics" of the 21st century by the World Health Organization, insofar as it is considered as one of the priority non-transmissible diseases due to the high morbidity and mortality related with their complications and the socioeconomic impact on public health systems in both developed and developing countries.

Diabetes can cause chronic complications in various organs of the body. Microvascular complications include complications in the foot (in diabetic foot that may progress to amputations), Kidney (chronic renal failure in an advanced stage may lead to the need for renal function replacement through dialysis or renal transplantation) and in the Eye (diabetic retinopathy is one of the main culprits of avoidable blindness in adults). Macrovascular complications can lead to acute myocardial infarction (AMI) and cerebrovascular accident (CVA), being an important cause of morbidity and mortality (Direção Geral Saúde (b), 2017).

The treatment of diabetes should have as main goal the implementation of measures aimed at the correction of lifestyles, in order to avoid the complications associated with the disease. Thus, pharmacological treatment must always be associated with non-pharmacological treatment. The Mediterranean diet, weight control and monitoring and increase of physical activity in a way adapted to the age and the health condition, in order to avoid sedentarism, are the basis of non-pharmacological treatment (Carvalho, Silva & Coelho, 2015), as it will be later explored.

Primary Health Care is essential in the prevention of this disease, through sensitization to behavioural change and/or adoption of healthy lifestyles, screening and early detection of potential cases of diabetes. Professionals in this area are important vectors of behaviour change in individuals with risk factors and in people with diabetes, in what refers to decision-making processes that allow them to self-control their lives (Figueiredo, 2017).

The professional practice of the nurse is implicit in all levels of prevention: in the prevention of the emergence of diseases through activities of promotion and protection of health (primary prevention); disease, and to treat it effectively in order to reverse it, cure it, alleviate or treat its severity (secondary prevention), and prevent disease progression or try to maintain the highest quality of life when process is considered irreversible (tertiary prevention).

Care for people with diabetes requires articulation between different levels of care, promoting multidisciplinarity and the participation of all institutions involved in this response.

NUTRITIONAL INTERVENTION

Nutritional intervention is fundamental to the treatment of type 1 and type 2 diabetes and in educating individual self-management ("Standards of Medical Care in Diabetes—2014," 2014).

The food selection and the adherence with the individualized food plan are the most challenging parts of the treatment for many diabetics (ADA, 2018b). The review by Hamdy & Barakatun-Nisak (2016), which included different studies, showed that the medical nutrition therapy improved glycemic control, weight loss promotion, and the reduction of the cardiovascular risk factors in individuals with diabetes. The reduction of carbohydrate load, selection of low glycemic index food, and balancing macronutrients revealed improved postprandial blood glucose levels. A selection of healthful dietary patterns, such as the Mediterranean diet or DASH diet, also had demonstrated to be beneficial in managing diabetes (Hamdy & Barakatun-Nisak, 2016).

The guidelines of the most important scientific organizations suggest:

- **Nutritionally Balanced Diet**
  - This diet reduces daily caloric intake (between 250 and 500 calories) to promote weight loss in overweight/obese adults.

- **Macronutrient Distribution**
  - Macronutrient distribution should be individualized - There is no single consensual dietary distribution of calories among fats, proteins and carbohydrates. Recommendations from different sources vary for lipids between 20 to 35%, for proteins between 15 to 30% and carbohydrates between 40 to 60%.

- **Eating Pattern**
  - Different eating patterns (based on personal preference, values and abilities) are acceptable for the management of type 2 diabetes and prediabetes.

- **Dietary Carbohydrate**
  - Food with a low GI value - carbohydrate intake from vegetables, whole grains, fruits, and dairy products, with an emphasis on foods higher in fibre and lower in glycemic load, is preferred over other sources like refined carbohydrates (processed grains, and starchy foods) and especially those containing added sugars. The prescription of a flexible insulin therapy program, an education plan on how to use carbohydrate counting and, in some cases, fat and protein gram estimation to determine mealtime insulin dosing, are recommended to improve glycemic control.

- **Dietary Fibre**
  - Foods with higher fibre (25-50g per day or 15-25 per 1000 Kcal).

- **Protein**
  - It is desirable to maintain protein intake below 15% of total daily calories (1.0 -1.5g/Kg body weight). Protein intake appears to increase insulin response without increasing plasma glucose concentrations (carbohydrate sources high in protein should be avoided when trying to treat or prevent hypoglycemia). Individuals with signs of kidney disease should consult a nephrologist before increasing protein intake.

- **Dietary Fat**
  - Data on the recommended total dietary fat content for people with diabetes are inconclusive. Reducing the percentage of fat (less than 35% of total daily calories), especially saturated (less than 7% of daily energy intake) and eating

foods rich in long-chain n-3 fatty acids, such as fatty fish (EPA and DHA) and nuts and seeds (ALA), is recommended to prevent or treat cardiovascular disease.

- **Supplements**
  - There is no clear evidence. However, many studies show the hypoglycemic effects of different bioactive compounds.

- **Alcohol**
  - Alcohol consumption without moderation may place people with diabetes at increased risk for hypoglycemia - no more than 1 drink (*e.g.* 150 mL wine) per day for women and 2 drinks for men (*e.g.* 300 mL wine). Individuals taking insulin or insulin secretagogues should pay special attention.

- **Sodium**
  - Consumption up to 2,3g/day (further restriction may be indicated for individuals with hypertension).

(ADA, 2018b; Hamdy & Barakatun-Nisak, 2016)

The consumption of complex carbohydrates (up to 60% of total calories) should be preferred to foods poor in fibre and with a low glycemic index, limiting the consumption of sucrose and other added sugars to no more than 10% of total energy (Clemente, Gallo, & Giorgini, 2018).

A 6-month randomized trial study suggests that a non-restrictive dietary intervention based on a Mediterranean or a low-fat diet in individuals with metabolic syndrome and type 1 diabetes could contribute to weight management, without significant differences between interventions for anthropometric and metabolic parameters (Fortin, Rabasa-Lhoret, Lemieux, Labonté, & Gingras, 2018).

The nutritional needs and preferences of each subject should, as far as possible, be attended for the success of the nutritional approach as part of a more complex intervention on the individual's lifestyle. Actually, an individualized food plan provided by a registered dietitian/nutritionist is indispensable for all people with different types of diabetes mellitus (type 1, type 2 or gestational) (ADA, 2018b).

Strong evidence supports the effectiveness of nutrition therapy provided by registered dietitian/nutritionist on:

- HbA1c with decreases up to 2.0% at 3 months, with ongoing nutrition therapy

support, decreases were maintained or improved long-term;
- Nutrition practice guideline should be integrated into the Nutrition Care Process (nutrition assessment, nutrition intervention, and nutrition monitoring and evaluation);
- The focus in individuals with type 2 diabetes is reducing energy intake; for individuals with type 1 diabetes is using carbohydrate counting to determine premeal insulin boluses;
- Medication use and quality of life;
- Importance of several initial encounters for assessment, intervention, and evaluation, and follow-up encounters for continued education and support (implementation of 3 to 6 encounters during the first 6 months with registered dietitian nutritionists);
- A minimum of one annual nutrition therapy follow-up encounter is also recommended;
- Individualized nutrition therapy implemented in collaboration with the individual.

(ADA, 2018a; Franz *et al.*, 2017)

Successful evaluation and diabetes management depend on beneficial interactions between the individual and the combined interventions of the care team (including a registered dietitian/nutritionist) who provide evidence-based, efficient nutrition therapy (ADA, 2018a; Franz *et al.*, 2017).

Future Perspectives in the Nutritional Intervention of Diabetes

The prevention and management of type 2 diabetes can be managed by precision nutrition, tailoring dietary interventions or recommendations to one or a combination of an individual's genetic background, metabolic profile, and environmental exposures. By integrating metabolomics, genomics, and gut microbiome technologies with big data analytics, precision nutrition has the potential to give personalized nutrition guidance for more efficient prevention and management of diabetes (Wang & Hu, 2018).

Significant novel nutritional therapeutic strategies have been proven to be an important tool in the development, onset and control of disease, mainly the discussion of how dietary interventions modulate the non-coding landscape in type 2 diabetes mellitus (Matboli *et al.*, 2018).

PHYSICAL ACTIVITY AND DIABETES

Some Evidence on Physical Activity Related to Diabetes

To address the benefits of physical activity in patients with Diabetes Mellitus, a search was conducted and some studies published in some databases were gathered.

According to Knuth (2009) in the study "Knowledge of adults on the role of physical activity in the prevention and treatment of diabetes and hypertension: a population-based study in the South of Brazil", it is possible to verify that knowledge about the physical activity in the prevention and treatment of diabetes and hypertension was associated with the independent variable. Knowledge can make a difference, scientific evidence of the importance of physical activity, both in the prevention and in delaying the onset of chronic diseases, are becoming more frequent and valued. However, the levels of general physical activity and in leisure, where the prevention benefits could be enhanced, in several parts of the world, are still very low. There is also evidence that population levels of physical activity are falling, especially among children and adolescents. The adoption of healthy lifestyles by individuals with Diabetes Mellitus demonstrates that health education and increased knowledge of the population's health help prevent this disease. The importance of the population's knowledge about the role of physical activity in the prevention of hypertension and diabetes is one of the possible ways to adopt a more active lifestyle to promote quality of life, increase health conditions and reduce palliative public expenditures with the treatment of these diseases. Even in cases of already ill individuals, it is known that strict control of blood glucose and blood pressure can reduce future complications with the natural course of these diseases.

In a study by Sartoreli & Franco (2003) entitled: "Trends of diabetes mellitus in Brazil: the role of nutritional transition", it has been discussed that it is possible to extract some information about the lifestyles and physical activity practiced by the population, and how these factors influence the disease. There is evidence that changes in lifestyle and associated with the frequent practise of physical activities, at least thirty minutes a day can act beneficially in the quality of life of the population and the burden of diseases to the public health system. This study clearly shows the benefits of physical activity and a healthy diet in reducing the incidence of disease cases as a form of prevention.

Finally, Guimarães & Takayanagui (2002) study on "Guidelines received from the health service by patients for the treatment of patients with type 2 diabetes mellitus", concludes about the importance that health professionals and users attribute to the prevention of the disease through physical activity. It states that it is necessary to know better the considerations of the individual with diabetes in relation to his/her treatment and to know the importance given to the practice of activities such as physical exercise and adherence to the food plan. It is possible to affirm that a more specific preparation of the entire health team is necessary, expanding their knowledge and thus allowing better adaptation of the guidelines to be provided to patients with this disease. Physical exercise with an adequate diet plan is also important and contribute significantly to recovery and improvements in the quality of life of the individual with the disease, and the treatment should not be based solely on a pharmacological intervention.

Known Benefits of Exercise for the Prevention and Minimization of Diabetes

Physical activity is very important for any individual since it is scientifically proven that physical inactivity is detrimental to health. Exercise helps in the improvement of bone density, muscular strength, body flexibility, motor and metabolic abilities, as well as cognitive function, mental health and social adjustment (Katzer, 2007). The low cost of physical practice, coupled with its non-pharmacological nature, further enhances its therapeutic utility. Physical activity plays an important role in the prevention of diabetes complications and in controlling glycemic levels. This is because it stimulates the pancreas to produce insulin that facilitates glucose transportation to cells. When exercising, the muscles need energy, increasing the use of glucose by preventing it from accumulating in the blood and increasing glycemia levels. In addition, it also decreases insulin resistance, lowers blood glucose levels during and after exercise, improves lipid profile, reduces hypertension; increases energy consumption, helps to lose weight and preserves muscle mass, increases strength and flexibility and improves the sense of well-being. Physical inactivity can lead to obesity, and excessive weight gain may contribute to the early onset of Diabetes Mellitus 2, while at the same time becoming an aggravating factor in metabolic control in young people already suffering from Diabetes Mellitus 1. Nevertheless, physical activity should be adjusted to the individual, according to their gender, age, capabilities and limitations, to avoid risks and optimize their benefits (Arrechea & Mercuri, 2001).

To prevent diseases, it is important to choose healthy eating habits and avoid sedentary lifestyles. Most of the benefits of physical activity in the treatment of type II diabetes are related to acute and chronic responses to insulin action in both aerobic and resistance exercises. It is important to emphasize the importance of monitoring by a professional in cases where the individual has diabetes, due to the risks that can occur. Therefore, it is normal and advisable for the professional to accompany the individual in the activities. Although physical activity is one of the key elements in the prevention and treatment of Type II diabetes, many people with this disease are less active or engage in irregular physical activity. It is fundamental to act in several areas: diet, exercise and medication, that is, the type II diabetes patient needs to make a lifestyle change. The treatment of type I diabetes, since the individuals are insulin-dependent, encompasses three fundamental aspects: adoption of an adequate diet, regular practice of physical activity and, of course, the administration of insulin. The goal of treatment is to keep the blood glucose level as close as possible to the values considered normal, so that they feel good and without any symptoms. Any physical activity can be beneficial for diabetics if well guided by professionals.

Types of Advisable Exercises for Diabetes

Aerobic, anaerobic or mixed exercises such as walking, swimming, cycling and dancing could be prescribed. With these exercises, it is possible to increase aerobic capacity, increase workload, decrease risk factors and improve hemodynamic response. Physical activity in this group should be practiced five to seven times per week, with workouts of twenty to forty minutes. These individuals, when practicing physical activity, should consider: measuring blood glucose levels before and after training, exercising lightly when the disease is imbalanced, reducing insulin doses on days of activity, taking a small meal before exercise to prevent hypoglycemia and maintain hydration. The practical recommendations for the practice of physical exercise for diabetics are:

• Wear comfortable socks and shoes;
• Keep foot care such as preventing athlete's foot;
• Avoid vigorous exercises that increase blood pressure;
• Do not exercise when the systolic pressure is greater than 180 mmHg.

The low and medium intensity long-term (aerobic) exercises are most indicated with an intensity corresponding to 50% of the maximum oxygen volume (Arrechea & Mercuri, 2001). These exercises improve glucose utilization. In the elderly, exercises for diabetics must be adapted because they have lower strength and muscle mass, so a good option will be choosing resistance exercise. In this type of exercise, a counterforce is exerted through a resistance, which increases the tension inside the muscle, delaying the consequences of ageing and improving glycemic control in the elderly (Santarém, 1999).

The practice of physical exercise corresponds to a better control of the blood glucose levels, since it causes an increase of the action of the insulin, increases the uptake of glucose by the muscle and increases the cellular sensitivity to the insulin. With this, there is often a decrease in the amount of medication, insulin and better control of diabetes.

According to the Diabetes Prevention Program (2012), there was a 58% reduction in the incidence of diabetes cases by stimulating a healthy diet and exercise.

OCCUPATIONAL THERAPY AND THE ROLE OF INTERVENTION IN THE PERSON WITH DIABETES

Diabetes Mellitus (DM) is considered a chronic-degenerative disease which can achieve both simple everyday activities and the most complex activities related to human occupation. The Occupational Therapist (OT) analyses the occupational performance of the subject, inserted in its context, and to optimize the functionality in the occupational areas. It should also include the multi-professional teams that provide care and treatment to the individual with DM, in order to promote a better quality of life for the dependent person, either with emotional support or through health education actions (Toscano, 2011).

Although some intervention strategies used in Occupational Therapy are shared between disciplines, their comprehensive goal of promoting occupational participation and their focus on activities such as unit analysis and intervention are unique within the diabetes treatment team (Pyatak *et al.*, 2018).

Several factors influence changes in the occupational performance of the individual with DM, such as lack of prevention, knowledge of the disease, post-diagnosis guidelines and care related to Daily Life Activities (DLA), Instrumental Daily Life Activities (IDLA), as well as the fragility of health services. In this sense, OT interventions focus on activity analysis, which deconstructs the requirements of an activity at the individual's level (sensory, cognitive and neuromuscular functions, social and process interaction skills, values and beliefs, and roles, habits and routines), the task (tools and resources required, physical space, social interaction, time and sequencing) and the environment (physical, social, cultural and temporal context).

Functional Consequences of Complications Associated with Diabetes

Diabetic neuropathies are characterized by a set of chronic peripheral neurological abnormalities (Almeida & Cruz, 2007) caused by diabetes and affecting mainly older people (National Institutes of Health and Care Excellence, 2015; Gooch & Podwall, 2004) burns or stinging pain, paraesthesia, hyperalgesia, loss of tactile sensitivity, allodynia, or severe pain that aggravates during the night period (Boulton, 2000). The American Diabetes Association (2005) states that these changes in sensitivity coupled with decreased blood circulation lead to an increased risk of developing foot ulcers and increased healing time.

The American Diabetes Association (2005) states that these changes in sensitivity coupled with decreased blood circulation lead to an increased risk of developing foot ulcers and increased healing time. These alterations in scarring may lead to the appearance of gangrene, the main cause of amputations in this population (Çakici, Fakkel, van Neck, Verhagen & Coert, 2016). That is, among some complications associated with DM is the diabetic foot, which is characterized by changes in neurological, vascular and infectious origin and constitutes a public health problem. Complications of the diabetic foot, if left untreated, may progress to the minor (foot) or major (thigh, leg or ankle) amputations, with important impact on functioning, disability, early retirement and increased morbidity.

The daily life of a diabetic person can represent a challenge for both the person and those close to him/her, since the condition of being diabetic and amputated affects life, drastically altering their daily life (Batista & Luz, 2012). In this case, OT aims at the training of the individual with diabetes, focusing on health education approach, on the general care that should be taken with the diabetic foot (hygiene, advising on the use of adequate footwear), as well as intervening in cases of amputation on the process of physical and functional rehabilitation of the individual associated with advising on the acquisition and training of assistive products (wheelchairs, prostheses, orthoses, bath and dressing aids), in order to facilitate functioning and functional mobility, for example transfers. It is possible for the OT to also intervene in the counselling of occupations, the adaptation of routines and activities and adjustment of the environment in the sense that it promotes greater independence in the tasks of daily life.

According to the National Institute for Health Care & Excellence (2015), neuropathies can manifest themselves in any organ or system, including the digestive tract, heart, and sex organs. There may also be presence of limb muscle weakness, carpal tunnel syndrome, limited range of motion, dizziness, osteomyelitis, deformities and depression (Çakici *et al.*, 2016), as well as changes in mobility and limitations in social participation (Blaum, Ofstedal, Langa, & Wray, 2003; Galer, Gianas, & Jensen, 2000).

Other studies have also shown that there is a direct correlation of neuropathy with other microvascular complications such as nephropathy, which can lead to renal failure, and diabetic retinopathy leading to decreased visual capacity and, in more serious cases, can lead to a total loss of vision (Birth, Pupe, Calvacanti, 2016).

Diabetic retinopathy is one of the main causes of avoidable blindness in the adult person, being considered as a major highlight in the disturbance of the individual's functionality in his daily activities with great impact on social and leisure activities. Therefore, the need for OT's intervention on and in the context, in the adaptation of the environment and of the task, complemented with the advice of assistive products, in the perspective of valuing the person's life history and in their significant activities and preserved performance skills. In addition to epidemiological surveillance, prevention practices and early diagnosis are essential.

In this way, the great impact that diabetes has on the functional capacity of the individual is perceived, which in the long term is reflected in a limitation of their participation and autonomy. In her review of the literature, Pyatak's (2010) citing Wallhagen (1999), confirms this idea by stating that, at any age, the client with diabetes undergoes a change in performance in all areas of occupation as a result of various modifications to which it is subject and the requirements of his/her environment.

For this reason, it is essential to intervene in the treatment of neuropathy and its consequences. Most of the literature refers to pharmacological treatment as the main method in the treatment of neuropathy. However, Çakici *et al.* (2016), in a study evaluating several types of pharmacological and non-pharmacological treatment, stated that TENS (transcutaneous electrical stimulation) and massage seem to obtain good results especially for the relief of painful symptoms. In addition, the same author refers to the importance of physical rehabilitation treatment in the prevention of muscle weakness and changes in coordination.

Moreover, regarding the changes in motor skills, Chiu *et al.* (2014) report how sensory, strength and coordination changes at the upper limb level can lead to difficulties in manual dexterity and fine motor skills. In the lower limbs, due to sensory changes (on contact with the floor), gait changes can be seen with the occurrence of imbalances and, in the most extreme cases, falls. For this reason, the implementation of a program of activities in occupational therapy for the training of these competences would be fundamental in the preservation of the same and, in this way, in the prevention of the emergence of the incapacities.

In a final note, we cannot fail to mention the intervention on cognitive decline. There is a strong correlation between diabetes and cognitive decline, especially among the older population associated with Alzheimer's dementia, vascular dementia and stroke. Studies related to diabetes and cognitive abilities show that in this population, a decline in episodic memory, executive functions, verbal fluency, working memory, processing speed, flexibility, and cognitive control are evident (Cholerton, Baker, Montine, & Craft, 2016). In this way, it is important to implement cognitive stimulation activities that work on these competencies in order to prevent their decline. In more severe cases, where there is already an advanced decline in cognitive functions, it is important to intervene in the adaptation of the activities, routines and the environment where they occur in order to allow the continuity of the person's autonomy. Activities and routines must be readjusted and adapted to maintain independence and safety, for basic and instrumental DLA. Examples of possible environmental changes are setting calendars at home, creating an agenda with the description of the person's routines, setting visual cues and identifying the rooms in the house, implementing assistive products for DLA, communication, caregiver supervision, security and safety. It is also important to train caregivers in how to assist in ADL, contribute to cognitive stimulation, and deal with periods of disorientation, psychotic outbreaks and aggression. At the behavioral level, it is important to explain the caregiver to avoid confrontation and communicational strategies to turn off a fixation.

Thus, it has been observed that controlling diabetes is complex and usually requires the person to modify their typical habits and routines related to taking medication, monitoring glucose, adhering to a regular exercise plan and implementing an adequate diet regime for maintaining optimal health, (Thompson, 2014) being essential the use of strategies and techniques of empowerment and self-management with OT support.

Empowerment in Diabetes

The concept of empowerment is considered one of the pillars that underpin the health promotion model that has been guiding health policies in different countries (Carvalho & Gastaldo, 2008). Empowerment is a collaborative, customer-centric approach, tailored to the fundamental realities of diabetes management, and is designed to help people discover and develop the inherent capacity to be responsible for their own lives (Funnel & Anderson, 2004) of interactive teaching designed to involve in the person the ability to solve problems in order to meet their cultural and psychosocial needs. The approach of the empowerment of the diabetic patient covers a set of measures that discuss technical and ethical ways of how the relationship between the person with diabetes and the health professionals who aim to improve the results in the self-management of the disease should be oriented (Lopes, 2015). Self-management education for diabetes is an essential basis for the empowerment approach and is necessary for the person to effectively manage diabetes and make decisions.

Goal setting within the empowerment approach is a five-step process that provides patients with the information and clarity they need to develop and achieve their diabetes and lifestyle goals (Anderson *et al.*, 1991): i) define the problem; ii) investigate the person's beliefs, thoughts and feelings that can support or hinder their efforts; iii) identify long-term goals for which work is to be done; iv) choose and commit to make a change of behavior; and v) evaluate the efforts and identify learning during the process.

Investing in transdisciplinary health promotion work can provide improved quality of life for people with diabetes to seek collective solutions and pave the way for a democratic exercise in decision-making, both in prevention and treatment (Bernini, 2017). The educational practice provides control of diabetes in addition to encouraging the participation of users in the management of the condition, increased empowerment and adherence to self-care practices, mainly for a healthy diet and practice of physical exercise. Other OT intervention strategies include the empowerment of the person with diabetes, sensory desensitization and adaptation of the environment, making it calm and relaxing at the time of insulin application and strategies for emotional regulation.

Self-management and Occupational Therapy

DM is a disease that requires continuous medical care with multifactor strategies for risk reduction, in addition to glycemic control. Educating the person for ongoing self-management and support is critical to prevent acute complications and minimize long-term risks in order to reduce complications resulting from the disease, reduce hospitalizations, and thus provide significant improvements in individuals' quality of life. Diabetes Self-management (DSM) has the potential to improve health-related quality of life, self-efficacy, functional difficulties as activities of daily living (ADL) and the performance of multiple domains of physical and mental health (Carvalho & António, 2018). Given that DSM is a classic example in which lifestyle adjustment is an important component of disease management, the expertise of occupational therapists in facilitating lifestyle changes is a promising resource in the development and implementation of more effective DSM interventions.

The intervention through the DSM focuses on behavioral and educational strategies aimed at producing weight loss, improving glycemic control, knowledge about diabetes, or reducing cardiovascular risk factors (Whittemore, 2006). OT services in the treatment of DM should offer a component of the person's education as a viable economic alternative to hospital care and a means to reduce future hospitalizations. The occupational therapist's goals in this program are to educate clients on the impact of physical activity and stress on diabetes management to address specific issues such as poor circulation and diabetic foot ulcers to provide information about relevant community resources and involve the person in control of the disease as an occupation in their daily routine.

Lorig and Holman (2003) developed a self-management intervention for chronic conditions that focus on skills development, such as problem-solving, decision making, action planning and self-adaptation (a strategy that allows people to customize an intervention for meet their needs). Much of the potential for improving health comes from the individual's ability to engage in DSM techniques in their daily lives, creating a lifestyle that promotes health and is sustainable in the long run. Intervention should include educational and skill-building elements, and allow customization through self-adaptation between occupation, participation and health (Pyatak, 2011).

Although DSM is not an area of practice within which occupational therapists traditionally work, it is a promising area of future growth for the profession. Studies on the role of occupational therapy in DSM are still limited, reflecting how infrequently occupational therapists treat this disorder as a primary diagnosis.

CONCLUDING REMARKS

Managing diabetes requires a change in lifestyle, whether it is improving eating habits, practicing physical activity, medication control, and self-care activities. The complications of the disease have an impact on the autonomy and independence of daily activities of the person, where it is necessary to intervene with a multi-professional approach centred on the person. However, the selection of treatment will depend on the stage of the disease and the individual's individual characteristics. Although there has been a growing number of studies on the subject in recent years, there is still a need to become better acquainted with mechanisms related to diabetes throughout the life cycle in order to give greater consistency to the recommendations and criteria for treatment and benefits short-term and long-term interventions.

CONSENT FOR PUBLICATION

Not applicable.

CONFLICT OF INTEREST

The author confirms that this chapter contents have no conflict of interest.

ACKNOWLEDGEMENTS

Declared none.

REFERENCES

Almeida, T., Cruz, S.C. (2007). Neuropatia diabética. *Revista Portuguesa de Medicina Geral e Familiar, 23*(5), 605-13.
[http://dx.doi.org/10.32385/rpmgf.v23i5.10409]

American Diabetes Association. (2018a). 3. Comprehensive Medical Evaluation and Assessment of

Comorbidities: *Standards of Medical Care in Diabetes-2018. Diabetes Care,* *41* (Suppl. 1), S28-S37. [http://dx.doi.org/10.2337/dc18-S003] [PMID: 29222374]

American Diabetes Association. (2018b). 4. Lifestyle Management: *Standards of Medical Care in Diabetes-2018. Diabetes Care,* *41* (Suppl. 1), S38-S50. [http://dx.doi.org/10.2337/dc18-S004] [PMID: 29222375]

American Diabetes Association. (2005). Diagnosis and Classification of Diabetes Mellitus. *Diabetes Care.,* (Suppl 1), s37-s42. [http://dx.doi.org/10.2337/diacare.28.suppl_1.S37] [PMID: 15618111]

American Diabetes Association. (2014). Standards of medical care in diabetes-2014. *Diabetes Care,* 37, (Suppl 1). Pp.S14–S80. [https://doi.org/10.2337/dc14-S014]

Anderson, R.M., Funnell, M.M., Barr, P.A., Dedrick, R.F., Davis, W.K. (1991). Aprender a capacitar os pacientes. *Diabetes Care,* *14*, 584-590. [http://dx.doi.org/10.2337/diacare.14.7.584] [PMID: 1914799]

Andrew, M.A. (1987). The occupational therapist's role in the management of diabetes. *Can. J. Occup. Ther.,* *54*(1), 11-15. [http://dx.doi.org/10.1177/000841748705400104] [PMID: 10280686]

dos Diabéticos de Portugal, A.P. (2012). Viver com a Diabetes.(3a ed.). Lisboa: Lidel Edições Técnicas, Lda.

Barreto, M., Kislaya, I., Gaio, V. (2017). Prevalência, conhecimento e controlo da diabetes em Portugal – resultados do Inquérito Nacional de Saúde com Exame Físico (INSEF 2015). *Boletim Epidemiológico Observações,* *6*(9), 34-38. Available at: http://hdl.handle.net/10400.18/4765

Batista, N.N., Luz, M.H. (2012). Vivências de pessoas com diabetes e amputação de membros. *Rev. Bras. Enferm.,* *65*(2), 244-250. [http://dx.doi.org/10.1590/S0034-71672012000200007] [PMID: 22911405]

Bernini, L. S., Barrile, S. R., Mangili, A. F., Arca, E. A., Correr, R., Ximenes, M. A., Gimenes, C. (2017). The impact of diabetes mellitus on the quality of life of patients of Primary Health Care *Cad. Bras. Ter. Ocup., São Carlos,* *25*(3), 533-541.

Boulton, A. J. (2000). The diabetic foot: a global view. *Diab/Metab Res Rev,* 16(S1), S2-S5. [https://doi.org/10.1002/1520-7560(200009/10)16:1+<::AID-DMRR105>3.0.CO;2-N] [PMID: 11054879]

Çakici, N., Fakkel, T.M., van Neck, J.W., Verhagen, A.P., Coert, J.H. (2016). Systematic review of treatments for diabetic peripheral neuropathy. *Diabet. Med.,* *33*(11), 1466-1476. [http://dx.doi.org/10.1111/dme.13083] [PMID: 26822889]

Carvalho, P. S., António, C. I. (2018). Sintomas psicopatológicos e vulnerabilidade ao estresse em uma amostra portuguesa de indivíduos com diabetes. *Revista Psicologia-Teoria e Prática,* 20(1).

Carvalho, S.R., Gastaldo, D. (2008). Promoção à saúde e empoderamento: uma reflexão a partir das perspectivas crítico-social pós-estruturalista. *Ciência & Saúde Coletiva* Rio de Janeiro.

Carvalho, S., Silva, T., Coelho, J. (2015). Contribuicões do tratamento não farmacológico para a Diabetes Mellitus tipo 2. Revista de Epidemiologia e Controle de Infecção *5*(2), 59-64.

Centers for Disease Control and Prevention. (2011). National diabetes fact sheet: national estimates and general information on diabetes and prediabetes in the United States, 2011 *Atlanta, GA: US Department of Health and Human Services, Centers for Disease Control and Prevention. 201*(1).

Chiu, H.Y., Hsu, H.Y., Kuo, L.C., Su, F.C., Yu, H.I., Hua, S.C., Lu, C.H. (2014). How the impact of median neuropathy on sensorimotor control capability of hands for diabetes: an achievable assessment from functional perspectives. *PLoS One,* *9*(4), e94452. [http://dx.doi.org/10.1371/journal.pone.0094452] [PMID: 24722361]

Cholerton, B., Baker, L.D., Montine, T.J., Craft, S. (2016). Type 2 diabetes, cognition, and dementia in older adults: toward a precision health approach. *Diabetes Spectr.,* *29*(4), 210-219.

[http://dx.doi.org/10.2337/ds16-0041] [PMID: 27899872]

Clemente, G., Gallo, M., Giorgini, M. (2018). Modalities for assessing the nutritional status in patients with diabetes and cancer. *Diabetes Res. Clin. Pract., 142*, 162-172
[http://dx.doi.org/10.1016/j.diabres.2018.05.039] [PMID: 29857095]

DGS - Direção Geral de Saúde. (2011). *Diagnóstico e Classificação da Diabetes Mellitus.* Norma da Direção Geral de Saúde.

DGS (b)- Direção Geral da Saúde. (2017). *Programa Nacional para a Diabetes 2017.* Lisboa, Portugal: Direção Geral da Saúde.

Figueiredo, M.H. (2017). Jornal Enfermeiro: Contextos, Competências e Necessidades em Enfermagem. Obtido de http://www.jornalenfermeiro.pt/opiniao/item/1490-formacao-dos-enfermeiros-para-a-diabetes.html

Fisher, J.D., Fisher, W.A., Amico, K.R., Harman, J.J. (2006). An information-motivation-behavioral skills model of adherence to antiretroviral therapy. *Health Psychol., 25*(4), 462-473.
[http://dx.doi.org/10.1037/0278-6133.25.4.462] [PMID: 16846321]

Fortin, A., Rabasa-Lhoret, R., Lemieux, S., Labonté, M.E., Gingras, V. (2018). Comparison of a Mediterranean to a low-fat diet intervention in adults with type 1 diabetes and metabolic syndrome: A 6-month randomized trial. *Nutr. Metab. Cardiovasc. Dis., 28*(12), 1275-1284.
[http://dx.doi.org/10.1016/j.numecd.2018.08.005] [PMID: 30459054]

Franz, M.J., MacLeod, J., Evert, A., Brown, C., Gradwell, E., Handu, D., Reppert, A., Robinson, M. (2017). Academy of nutrition and dietetics nutrition practice guideline for type 1 and type 2 diabetes in adults: Systematic review of evidence for medical nutrition therapy effectiveness and recommendations for integration into the nutrition care process. *J. Acad. Nutr. Diet., 117*(10), 1659-1679.
[http://dx.doi.org/10.1016/j.jand.2017.03.022] [PMID: 28533169]

Funnell, M.M., Anderson, R.M. (2004). Empowerment and self-management of diabetes. *Clin. Diabetes, 22*(3), 123-127.
[http://dx.doi.org/10.2337/diaclin.22.3.123]

Galer, B.S., Gianas, A., Jensen, M.P. (2000). Painful diabetic polyneuropathy: epidemiology, pain description, and quality of life. *Diabetes Res. Clin. Pract., 47*(2), 123-128.
[http://dx.doi.org/10.1016/S0168-8227(99)00112-6] [PMID: 10670912]

Gooch, C., Podwall, D. (2004). The diabetic neuropathies. *Neurologist, 10*(6), 311-322.
[http://dx.doi.org/10.1097/01.nrl.0000144733.61110.25] [PMID: 15518597]

Guimarães, F., Takayanagui, A. (2002). Orientações recebidas do serviço de saúde por pacientes para o tratamento do portador de *diabetes mellitus* tipo. *Rev. Nutr., 1*, 37-44.
[http://dx.doi.org/10.1590/S1415-52732002000100005]

Hamdy, O., Barakatun-Nisak, M-Y. (2016). Nutrition in Diabetes. *Endocrinol. Metab. Clin. North Am., 45*(4), 799-817.
[http://dx.doi.org/10.1016/j.ecl.2016.06.010] [PMID: 27823606]

Katzer, J.I. (2007). *Diabetes Mellitus tipo II e atividade física. Revista Digital. Buenos Aires, nº113. Acedido a 9 de dezembro de 2015 em.*http://www.efdeportes.com/efd 113/diabetes-mellitus-e-atividade-fisica.htm

Knuth, A.G., Bielemann, R.M., Silva, S.G., Borges, T.T., Del Duca, G.F., Kremer, M.M., Hallal, P.C., Rombaldi, A.J., Azevedo, M.R. (2009). Conhecimento de adultos sobre o papel da atividade física na prevenção e tratamento de diabetes e hipertensão: estudo de base populacional no Sul do Brasil. *Cad. Saude Publica, 25*(3), 513-520.
[http://dx.doi.org/10.1590/S0102-311X2009000300006] [PMID: 19300840]

Lopes, A.A.F. (2015). Care and Empowerment: the construction of the subject responsible for his own health in the experience of diabetes. *Saude Soc., 24*(2), 486-500.
[http://dx.doi.org/10.1590/S0104-12902015000200008]

Lorig, K.R., Holman, H. (2003). Self-management education: history, definition, outcomes, and mechanisms.

Ann. Behav. Med., 26(1), 1-7.
[http://dx.doi.org/10.1207/S15324796ABM2601_01] [PMID: 12867348]

Mercuri, N., Arrechea, V. (2001). Atividade física e diabetes mellitus. *Diabetes Clínica, 5*(2), 347-349. Available at: http://www.saudeemmovimento.com.br/revista/artigos/diabetes_clinica/v5n5_exercicio.pdf

Matboli, M., Shafei, A., Ali, M., Kamal, K.M., Noah, M., Lewis, P., Habashy, A., Ehab, M., Gaber, A.I., Abdelzaher, H. (2018). Emerging role of nutrition and the non-coding landscape in type 2 diabetes mellitus: A review of literature. *Gene, 675*, 54-61.
[http://dx.doi.org/10.1016/j.gene.2018.06.082] [PMID: 29960068]

Nascimento, Pupe Calvacanti. (2016). Diabetic neuropathy *Rev Dor. São Paulo, 17*(1), 46-51.

National Institute for Health Care & Excellence (2015). Type 2 diabetes in adults: management (NG28). Available at https://www.nice.org.uk/guidance/ng28

Pyatak, E.A. (2011). The role of occupational therapy in diabetes self-management interventions. *OTJR (Thorofare, N.J.), 31*(2), 89-96.
[http://dx.doi.org/10.3928/15394492-20100622-01]

Pyatak, E.A., Carandang, K., Vigen, C.L.P., Blanchard, J., Diaz, J., Concha-Chavez, A., Sequeira, P.A., Wood, J.R., Whittemore, R., Spruijt-Metz, D., Peters, A.L. (2018). Occupational therapy intervention improves glycemic control and quality of life among Young adults with diabetes: the resilient, empowered, active living with diabetes (REAL diabetes) randomized controlled trial. *Diabetes Care, 41*(4), 696-704.
[http://dx.doi.org/10.2337/dc17-1634] [PMID: 29351961]

Santarém, J.M. (1999). Treinamento de força e potência. *O Exercício: Preparação Fisiológica, Avaliação Médica, Aspectos Especiais e Preventivos, 3550.* São Paulo: Ed. Atheneu.

Sartorelli, D., Franco, L. (2003). Tendências do diabetes mellitus no Brasil: o papel da transição nutricional. *Cad. Saude Publica, 19*, 29-36.
[http://dx.doi.org/10.1590/S0102-311X2003000700004]

Thompson, M. (2014). Occupations, habits, and routines: perspectives from persons with diabetes. *Scand. J. Occup. Ther., 21*(2), 153-160.
[http://dx.doi.org/10.3109/11038128.2013.851278] [PMID: 24215481]

Toscano, R.C.C. (2011). *Terapia Ocupacional: Uma Contribuição Ao Paciente Diabético.* Rio de Janeiro: Ed. Rubia.

Wang, D.D., Hu, F.B. (2018). Precision nutrition for prevention and management of type 2 diabetes. *Lancet Diabetes Endocrinol., 6*(5), 416-426.
[http://dx.doi.org/10.1016/S2213-8587(18)30037-8] [PMID: 29433995]

Whittemore, R. (2006). Behavioral interventions for diabetes self-management. *Nurs. Clin. North Am., 41*(4), 641-654, viii.
[http://dx.doi.org/10.1016/j.cnur.2006.07.014] [PMID: 17059979]

Wray, L.A., Ofstedal, M.B., Langa, K.M., Blaum, C.S. (2005). The effect of diabetes on disability in middle-aged and older adults. *J. Gerontol. A Biol. Sci. Med. Sci., 60*(9), 1206-1211.
[http://dx.doi.org/10.1093/gerona/60.9.1206] [PMID: 16183964]

CHAPTER 7

Celiac Disease and Modern Society

Catarina Lobão[1], Vânia Ribeiro[2], Rui Gonçalves[1] and Hugo Neves[1]

[1] *Nursing School of Coimbra, UICISA:E - Health Sciences Research Unit: Nursing, Coimbra, Portugal*

[2] *School of Health Sciences & ciTechCare - Center for Innovative Care and Health Technology, Polytechnic of Leiria, Portugal*

Abstract: Celiac Disease is a serious autoimmune disorder that can emerge in genetically predisposed persons where the ingestion of gluten could damage the small intestine. It can develop at any age and if left untreated, it can lead to severe health problems. Celiac disease has a hereditary component and when a celiac person eats gluten (a protein found in wheat, barley and rye), the body begins an immune response that leads to damage the small fingerlike projections (villous) of the small intestine, avoiding the proper absorption of nutrients into the body. In this chapter, we intend to present a brief review of the literature that has been produced, following the new perspectives on celiac disease approach. We present a brief description of recent advances in the celiac disease diagnosis, treatment and gluten-free diet.

Keywords: Barriers, Celiac Disease, Future Perspectives, Literacy.

INTRODUCTION

Celiac Disease (CD) is a systemic life-long gluten-sensitive autoimmune disorder induced by dietary gluten peptides found in rye, wheat and barley and is classified as one of the most common diseases (Gujral, Freeman, & Thomson, 2012; Kang, Kang, Green, Gwee, & Ho, 2013). It occurs in people who are genetically susceptible to ingestion of gluten which leads to mucosal damage of small intestine, with these patients potentially presenting gastrointestinal symptoms, extraintestinal symptoms or even no signs of any symptom. Classical symptoms could include diarrhea, steatorrhea and weight loss due to malabsorption, but an expressive part of the CD patients could present anemia osteoporosis, dermatitis herpetiformis, neurological and dental problems (extraintestinal or atypical symptoms).

* **Corresponding author Catarina Lobão:** Nursing School of Coimbra, UICISA:E - Health Sciences Research Unit: Nursing, Coimbra, Portugal; Tel: +351239802850/239487200; E-mail: catarinalobao@esenfc.pt

Samuel Honório, Marco Batista, Helena Mesquita & Jaime Ribeiro (Eds.)

Most patients with CD carry one of two major histocompatibility complex class II molecules (HLA-DQ2 or –DQ8) required to present gluten peptides in a manner that activates an antigen-specific T cell response. Although DQ2 or DQ8 is a major factor in the genetic predisposition to celiac disease most of the positive people never develop CD despite daily exposure to a gluten diet (Therrien & Kelly, 2018). Environmental factors and genetic factors required for the loss of immune tolerance to gluten diets are still unknown, but we know that the timing of initial gluten intake plays an important role, as well as the coexisting gastrointestinal infections or direct damage to the intestinal-epithelial barrier.

Ka *et al.* (2014) and Therrien & Kelly (2018), proposed that the loss of immune tolerance to the peptide antigens (from de gluten dietary) derived from prolamins in wheat (gliadin), rye (secalin) and barley (hordein) is the central abnormality of CD. As reported by Therrien and Kelly (2018), the human proteases could not decompose those peptides and persist intact in the small intestinal lumen stimulating interleukin-15 production by dendritic cells, macrophages and intestinal epithelial cells, which then stimulate intraepithelial lymphocytes, leading to epithelial damage. Cytotoxic T lymphocytes induced cell death, tissue remodeling with villous atrophy and subsequent antigliadin and anti-transglutaminase antibody production.

CD has been kept in the dark for a decade as a known child disease and only now has received a greater understanding of its prevalence, diagnosis and pathogenesis. The variability of the clinical picture of CD creates a spectrum with different forms as a result of the villous atrophy and hypertrophy of the intestinal crypts. There is no formal classification but Gujral *et al.* (2012), Kang *et al.* (2013), and Therrien & Kelly (2018) divided it into common subgroups: i) classic; ii) atypical; iii) silent; iv) nonresponsive; and v) refractory. The classic form emerges with typical symptoms as well as diarrhea, weight loss, abdominal pain and discomfort, and weakness. The atypical form presents with deficiency states (*e.g.* iron deficiency) or extraintestinal manifestations (*e.g.* fatigue, liver enzymes growing, infertility) and this form is likely to account for the largest number of patients with a CD diagnosis. Silent forms evidence serologic and histologic without any evident symptoms or signs. The nonresponsive form appears when clinical symptoms and laboratory abnormalities recur after gluten withdrawal or while the patient is on a gluten-free diet. The refractory form of CD defines the persistence of clinical symptoms and histological abnormalities after 6 months on a strict gluten-free diet and in the exclusion of other evident causes (Gujral *et al.*, 2012; Kang *et al.*, 2013; Therrien & Kelly, 2018).

CD is a life-long disorder, and if left untreated, it is associated with increased morbidity and mortality, and since 1970, the European Society of Paediatric

Gastroenterology highlights the criteria for the CD diagnosis in children based on three biopsies before and after a gluten-free diet.

Today's approach has been modified by the introduction of highly sensitive and specific serologic tests. The initial evaluation of CD is based on a combination of positive CD-specific serological tests, histological findings from intestinal biopsy, CD-predisposing gene encoding HLA DQ2 or DQ8, medical and family history of CD, and clinical and histological response to a gluten-free diet (Gujral *et al.*, 2012).

EPIDEMIOLOGY

Generally, the CD diagnosis is based on the presence of a predisposing genetic factor, human leukocyte antigen (HLA) DQ2/8, with positive biopsy and serological antibodies upon gluten contained diet. For several years, CD was considered a childhood disease mainly among white Europeans. Today, we know that CD is a common genetic disorder in many countries, with a uniform prevalence, slightly more likely in women, and maybe diagnosed at any age, with a first large peak period of presentation around the age of 6 to 7 years and a second large peak in the fourth and fifth lifetime decades (Therrien & Kelly, 2018). Geographic and temporal variation in the incidence of CD is a direct result of the effects of nutritional practices on the risk and severity of CD (Rewers, 2005), and be of great public health significance.

The available data suggest that CD incidence is increasing and is more common in some areas than earlier identified. The changes in diet habits, particularly in gluten consumption as well as in infant feeding patterns are probably the main factors that can account for these new trends in CD epidemiology (Ka *et al.*, 2014). The rapid increase in wheat intake in recent decades in countries that commonly produced gluten-free cereals like rice, maize, sorghum, and millet, is one of the main causes associated with the changes in the CD geographical variation.

Gujral *et al.* (2012) stated that the world distribution of CD seems to have followed the wheat consumption and the migratory flows with its prevalence being underestimated in the past. Following the same reasoning, the specialty literature suggests that many people may have a genetic predisposition to CD but the clinical presentation only occurs in the presence of gluten dietary.

Around the world, in most countries the CD prevalence is unknown and, when it exists, it is based on different reference sources (*e.g.* serology, biopsy, the two combined and with a response to gluten challenge). Among the factors that denote a higher risk for CD, researchers point out that the most important is family history, as the overall prevalence of CD is highly dependent on the HLA DQ2/DQ8 typing and gluten consumption.

The reasons for these global changes are truly unclear but have to do with changes in the quality and quantity of ingested gluten. Although the incidence of clinical diagnosis of CD cases is increasing, still the larger part of the "celiac iceberg" remains undetected (Ka *et al.*, 2014).

This is the overall CD scenario between European/North American countries and Asian/African and Middle East countries, the diagnosis rate is still very low and "submerged in an ocean of malnutrition". The efficacy of the CD case finding is poor, with more than 50% of the cases remaining undiagnosed. In this context, this study highlighted the need to assess the efficiency of new screening strategies.

The lack of consistent epidemiological studies aiming to clarify the role of all factors as well as the measure of the national prevalence of CD will play a strategical role in increasing the awareness of CD, enhancing appropriate screening, diagnosis, and redefinition of treatment guidelines.

LITERACY IN CELIAC DISEASE

Sources and Barriers

Health literacy can be defined as the "degree to which individuals have the capacity to obtain, process, and understand basic health information and services needed to make appropriate health decisions" (Institute of Medicine Committee on Health, 2004). This couldn't be accurate for people with celiac disease (PwCD) as, in order to prevent complications in celiac disease, they depend on high levels of literacy in order to manage a healthy life based on informed decision-making. PwCD require knowledge regarding the ingredients that compose the food they are eating, as well as the risk of cross-contact and how to reduce it.

However, in spite of this requirement, Silvester, Weiten, Graff, Walker, and Duerksen (2016) have found that individuals who believe to follow a Gluten-Free Diet (GFD) do not identify these foods correctly. Sources referred and considered useful by these individuals include cookbooks, internet, patient advocacy groups and other persons with the same condition, whereas family physicians were, not only the second least used source, but also referred to as the least helpful in regard to GFD (Silvester *et al.*, 2016; Zarkadas *et al.*, 2013). This underlines the need to develop strategies to disseminate knowledge to primary care physicians and nurses, transforming these professionals into a valuable resource by reducing health costs and increasing proximity. The use of apps may help reduce this barrier (Ventola, 2014) and make PwCD understand the valuable resource of primary care health professionals.

In children, gluten-free diet adherence has been increasing from ten years to present (Czaja-Bulsa & Bulsa, 2018), with peer acceptance clearly decreasing as the main barrier, which could be related to the success of public awareness on this condition. The same authors relate the main problem regarding adherence to a GFD in this population to the absence of symptoms after consumption of food containing gluten. Strategies to help these children and teenagers understand the negative impact of not following a GFD should be developed to optimize adherence. Gamification as a health promotion strategy may have a positive impact, with goal setting with reward and incentive, self-monitoring, and focus on past success as some of the behavior changing techniques more commonly used in other apps and with potential impact (Edwards *et al.*, 2016).

Associations and Foundations

Celiac associations have been contributing to a better quality of life for PwCD. With globalization, traveling to a foreign country may increase difficulty to adhere to a GFD. Many countries worldwide have policies to protect PwCD, with the national associations being a good source of information. As such, if thinking of traveling abroad, consulting a national association website (Table **1**) may help understand where to find GFD food, as well as restaurants certified to respect their needs.

Table 1. Associations and Foundations worldwide

Associations Worldwide	
Association of European Celiac Societies (AOECS): www.aoecs.org	Luxembourg: www.alig.lu
Andorra: www.celiacsandorra.org	Malta: coeliacassociationmalta.org
Austria: www.zoeliakie.or.at	Mexico: www.acelmex.org.mx
Australia: www.coeliac.org.au	Netherlands: www.glutenvrij.nl
Bermuda: Phone – 1.441.232.0264 (Coeliac Support Group of Bermuda)	New Zealand: www.coeliac.org.nz
Brazil: www.acelbra.org.br/english/index.php	Norway: www.ncf.no
Canada: www.celiac.ca	Pakistan: www.celiac.com.pk/index.php
Celiac Youth of Europe: www.cyeweb.eu	Panama: www.acepa.blogspot.com
Croatia: www.celijakija.hr	Paraguay: www.fupacel.org.py
Cyprus: www.cypruscoeliac.org	Poland: www.celiakia.pl

(Table 1) cont.....

Associations Worldwide	
Czech Republic: www.celiak.cz/en	Portugal: www.celiacos.org.pt
Denmark: www.coeliaki.dk	Russia (St. Petersburg): celiac.spb.ru
El Salvador: http://celiacos-el-salvador.blogspot.com/	Saudi Arabia: www.saudi-celiac.com/main
Estonia: www.tsoliaakia.ee	Slovenia: drustvo-celiakija.si
Finland: www.keliakialiitto.fi	Slovakia: www.celiakia.sk
France: www.afdiag.fr	Spain: www.celiacos.org
Germany: www.dzg-online.de	Spain (Catalunya): celiacscatalunya.org
Greece: www.coeliac.gr	Sweden: celiaki.se
Hungary: www.coeliac.hu/tiki-index.php	Switzerland: www.zoeliakie.ch
Ireland: www.coeliac.ie	Turkey: www.colyak.org.tr
India: www.celiacsocietyrajasthan.com	U.A.E.: www.glutenfreeuae.com
Italy: www.celiachia.it	Ukraine: www.celiac-ukraine.com
Israel: www.celiac.org.il	United Kingdom: www.coeliac.org.uk
Japan: www.foodallergy.jp	United Sates of America: celiac.org
Lebanon: www.lebaneseceliacs.org	Uruguay: www.acelu.org
Lithuania: www.begliuteno.lt	

Source: https://celiac.org/gluten-free-living/global-associations-and-policies/associations-around-the-world/

Cookbooks and Recipes

One major issue identified by PwCD relates to the taste and price of gluten-free food (Czaja-Bulsa & Bulsa, 2018). This can be a huge handicap as taste is more and more present in our days, with many culinary programs on television, outdoor food and restaurant advertisements identifying the importance of flavor. This poses a huge challenge, with the need to achieve a balance between GFD and avoid nutrient excess or deficiencies (Bascunan, Vespa, & Araya, 2017). Cooking at home may be a safe place to avoid eating food that underwent cross-contamination. Not only that but also the opportunity to improve flavor and personalize the diet may help adhere to a GFD. Many recipes and cookbooks may be available in local bookstores, and in national celiac associations websites and foundations, as well as Facebook® group pages. It is important for the healthcare professional to understand the importance given by the person to flavor and their preferences when having a GFD, thus improving quality of life.

Apps and Websites

The use of apps and games have become a reality in healthcare practice. Although this may be an opportunity to achieve a broader audience, there are certain dangers when selecting a specific app, such as privacy and quality of information.

Social media may also be another source of information to which healthcare professionals should be aware, especially with the population of young people that value information shared on social media which is thus transforming the role of social environment as a potential relevant resource (Levin-Zamir & Bertschi, 2018).

Social media can also be a relevant source of information to the healthcare professional, with some studies identifying patient-reported outcomes through analysis of the number of "likes" on Facebook® celiac groups, to understand which information PwCD value more (Park, Harris, Khavari, & Khosla, 2014).

Other websites and apps (Table **2**) provide information regarding types of food that are gluten-free. It is becoming very common the use of websites and apps in order to help understand what type of food is appropriate for PwCD. As such, the role of healthcare professionals is to develop competencies regarding the analysis of the tools available to guarantee the appropriation of the information to the needs of PwCD. Although most of these tools are of American origin, this may constitute an opportunity for app developers of other countries to adapt them to their culture, language and reality, providing better information in native language and culture.

Table 2. List of apps and respective websites

Apps	Website
Find Me Gluten-free	findmeglutenfree.com
Gluten-Free Marketplace 2.0	https://celiac.org/marketplace/gf-products/
AllergyEats	allergyeats.com
Gluten-free Restaurant Cards	celiactravel.com
Fooducate Healthy Weight Loss & Calorie Counter	fooducate.com
The Gluten-free Scanner	scanglutenfree.com
Is That Gluten-free?	gardenbaysoftware.com
Sift Food Labels	siftfoodlabels.com
ShopWell Diet, Allergy Scanner	shopwell.com
Celiac Disease, Wheat and Gluten	recoverybull.com
mySymptoms Food Diary	skygazerlabs.com

Source: https://www.glutenfreeliving.com/gluten-free-foods/shopping-gluten-free/top-10-gluten-free-apps/

Labeling

Labeling is one of the most important sources of information to PwCD.

Understanding food labeling is one of the most fundamental skills to develop in someone who suffers from this condition in order to adhere to a GFD (Muhammad, Reeves, Ishaq, Mayberry, & Jeanes, 2017; Zarkadas *et al.*, 2013).

Table 3. Allowed, dangerous and forbidden foods.

Allowed	Dangerous	Forbidden
Flour, starch and derivatives of carob, arrowroot, rice, potato, potato starch, manioc (and sprinkle of), corn, millet, quinoa, sorghum, teff, buckwheat, *etc.*	Cornbread	Flour and starch of:
Fruits and vegetables	Industrial cheese	• Wheat and varieties
Legumes (chickpeas, beans, lentils, *etc.*)	Creamy or yogurts with fruit pieces	• Rye
Oilseeds (nuts, almond, hazelnut, *etc.*)	Chocolate, malted or aromatized milk	• Barley
Seeds (sesame, sunflower, linseed, *etc.*)	Processed meat (minced meat, sausages, hamburgers, meatballs)	• Oats
Fat free, skimmed and half skimmed simple milk	Pre-cooked, frozen and ultra-frozen products	Malt and malt extract
Fresh and creamy cheese	Canned products, pâtés	Bread, bakery and confectionery products
Natural and flavored yogurts	Delicatessen products (ham, sausages, *etc.*)	Cookies and biscuits
Meat	Soy products (hamburgers, sausage, sauce)	Pasta
Fish	Cooking broth	Cereal yogurts
Eggs	Industrial sauces (ketchup, mayonnaise, mustard, chutney)	Pudding
Seafood	Curry	Packaged soups
Sugar, honey and molasses	Vinegar	Breaded products
Homemade jam and marmalade	Instant dessert	Oilcakes
Salt	Commercial ice creams	Pizza
Olive oil and vegetable oil	Commercial fruit jams	Lasagna, cannelloni, ravioli
Pure spices	Chocolate tablet or powder	Beer
Aromatic herbs	Crystalized/syrup fruit	Wheat, rye, barley, oats
Dry fresh biological yeast	Gelatins	Cereals
Water, tea and infusions	Dry figs	Forbidden cereals starch
Nectars, natural and sparkling fruit juices	Fresh cream	Starch (from an unknown origin)
Wine, Port, champagne, distilled drinks (whisky, rum, vodka)	Butter and margarines	Modified starch (from an unknown origin)
Pure coffee/decaffeinated, expresso	Industrial lard	Food fibers (from an unknown origin)
Glucose, glucose syrup	Flavored packaged french fries	Hydrolyzed wheat protein (from an unknown origin)
Dextrin, dextrose	Concentrates and powdered juices	Food additives of E-14XX group
Maltodextrin or malt dextrin	Glacé (powdered sugar)	
Sorbitol, maltitol, soy lecithin, inulin	Chemical powdered yeast	
Yeast		
All E-XXX food additives with the exception of E-14XX group		

To read a label, it is important for the PwCD to check for a gluten-free label, a list of allergens and obvious ingredients (Table **3**). It is also important to check for hidden or questionable ingredients and check a dietitian in case of any doubt.

Likewise, some apps have also been developed to aid in identifying which ingredients may be present in the label potentially with gluten. Supermarket suppliers, as well as policymakers should consider this increasing reality and adhere and develop policies for a better labeling of products. These strategies may help and assure PwCD in their quest to a GFD and a better quality of life.

Celiac Disease in the Elderly

Celiac Disease is not an age-related condition. In spite of not being usually related to the elderly, it is interesting to see that around 25% of first diagnosis occur in the seventh decade (Cappello, Morreale, & Licata, 2016). This is an important fact as, not only it highlights how sub-diagnosis of the disease might potentially occur in the present, but also that it is also a problem to be tackled in today's modern society as a serious health condition. First diagnosis in these ages may indicate that the disease is becoming symptomatic and complications may be worse due to longer exposure to gluten (Cappello *et al.*, 2016).

Adherence to a GFD may be a difficult task when we approach a population that has been eating food with gluten for decades. As most tools to help PwCD are targeted to a younger audience, this underlines the need to develop strategies to optimize communication and dissemination of knowledge in this population, focused on understanding what types of products are gluten-free, however, above all, how to avoid cross-contamination. Capacitation of the family relatives, more specifically children and grandchildren, as well as dissemination of this knowledge in senior institutions, such as nursing homes, may prove to be interventions that optimize adherence to a GFD.

Another important characteristic of this population relates to their cultural and spiritual beliefs that may impact a strict GFD. An example of this characteristic has been reported by Guiraldes and Gutierrez (1988) where the official body of the Catholic Church recommends taking wine as an alternative to the holy communion wafer, or a tiny fragment of the wafer or none at all. Also, the nutritional requirements of the elderly may lead to a different type of diet. Some studies indicate that a GFD may improve bone mineral density, but doesn't relate well to an increase in bone mass, indicating that this population may be more prone to osteoporosis and fractures (Cappello *et al.*, 2016). Other problems, such as the increased risk of cardiovascular diseases, refractory celiac disease, malignancy, are some of the complications mentioned in the literature, mostly due to the change in the absorption of medication (Cappello *et al.*, 2016).

TREATMENT OVERVIEW

Gluten-free Diet

A gluten-free diet is characterized by a combination of naturally occurring gluten-free foods with gluten-free substitutes for cereal-based foods and currently is the only acceptable therapeutic option for celiac disease (Ciacci *et al.*, 2015; Stein & Katz, 2017).

Gluten-free foods may contain until 20 mg gluten per Kg of total food, consisting of ingredients that do not contain wheat (all Triticum species, such as durum wheat, Khorasan wheat and spelt, barley, rye, oats or their crossbred varieties). This diet improves clinical manifestations, prevents bone disease, autoimmune conditions, and non-malignant and malignant complications (Stein & Katz, 2017).

Since the only restriction is gluten exclusion, the diet can be based on personal food choices. However, this diet may lead to nutrient imbalance, resulting in an improper nutritional quality (Vici, Belli, Biondi, & Polzonetti, 2016).

Nowadays, there are contrasting data about the nutritional adequacy of a gluten-free diet. Some diets adopted by celiac patients have low fiber content, being composed of starches and refined flours and with high sugar and fat contents. The gluten-free diets are also frequently poor in micronutrient like vitamins D, B12, folate and minerals, namely calcium, magnesium, iron and zinc (Vici *et al.*, 2016). To optimize the therapeutic approach in celiac patients, dietitians/nutrition professionals should evaluate the nutritional quality of diets and develop educational strategies (Vici *et al.*, 2016).

A study with 99 patients on a gluten-free diet was associated with a relevant chance of healing intestinal lesion and correction of specific body compositional. This study demonstrated that with the dietary compliance, the rates of mucosal remission (Marsh 0) and response (Marsh 0/1) improved considerably through the (5) years (Newnham, Shepherd, Strauss, Hosking, & Gibson, 2016).

In a Mediterranean diet, in a study that compares the eating habits between celiac patients and healthy individuals, it was verified that celiacs consumed more processed red meat, potatoes and fruit than healthy individuals. The Italian Mediterranean Index was significantly lower in celiac than in healthy individuals. Celiac patients should be encouraged to adjust their food choices to the recommended Mediterranean Diet in order to improve their nutritional status and protect against noncommunicable diseases in a long term (Morreale *et al.*, 2018).

To be successful, a gluten-free diet should be based on a variety of different cereals/starch sources that can include rice, maize, cassava, soy, potato, beans, buckwheat groats (also known as kasha), gluten-free oats, quinoa, sorghum, millet, amaranth, arrowroot, teff, flax, chia and nut flours. Choosing processed foods should also consider the high sugar and fat content that many products may contain. Gluten-free meals should be carefully prepared in order to avoid cross-contamination and to guarantee the balance of macro and micronutrients in patients' meals, privileging foods with lower sugar and fat content.

Although gluten-free diet is the basis of treatment, new therapeutic strategies are required because not all patients reach histological remission. Some of them are presented in the next section.

Study Therapies and Future Perspectives

Several treatments directed to different pathogenic targets of celiac disease have been developed in the last years, namely:

- Gluten removal of the hybridize species of *Triticum aestivum* – due to the lack of the genes encoding the immunogenic gluten-derived peptides (Stein & Katz, 2017).
- Gluten modification to produce non-immunogenic gluten - modifying gluten to make gliadin nontoxic using enzymatic or genetic manipulation of grains to reduce their immunogenicity and its content of toxic epitopes has benefits for the pharmacological treatments. The immunogenicity is reduced by enzymatic or genetic manipulation of grains (Jouanin, Boyd, Visser, & Smulders, 2018).
- Gluten replacement - using grains that do not contain immunogenic peptides like sorghum, is safe for consumption by patients with celiac disease (Stein & Katz, 2017).
- Enzymatic treatment of the flour - Hydrolyze immunogenic gluten peptides by sourdough *lactobacilli* and *fungal* proteases to obtain hydrolyzed wheat flour for the formulation of baked foods (Heredia-Sandoval, Valencia-Tapia, Calderón de la Barca, & Islas-Rubio, 2016).
- Probiotics - *lactobacilli* are able to hydrolyze the proline and glutamine-rich gluten peptides and reduced their toxicity, as well as protect the intestinal epithelium from damage induced by gliadin (Stein & Katz, 2017).

Other treatments in developing are based on modulation of intestinal permeability, regulation of the adaptive immune response and endoluminal therapies to degrade gluten in the intestinal lumen (Vaquero, Rodríguez-Martín, León, Jorquera, & Vivas, 2018), oral enzyme supplementation, larazotide acetate to prevent absorption of the gliadin peptides, synthetic polymers, reducing cytokine production, tTG2 inhibitors and vaccines (Stein & Katz, 2017).

CONCLUDING REMARKS

Despite the advances observed we must emphasize the important role that healthcare professionals have with the celiac person through scheduled or spontaneous enlightenment sessions on illness, eating or associated co-morbidities. Because it is an increasingly well-known and studied disease, this urges the need for greater social awareness, allowing the person with celiac disease to have a better quality of life, by bringing their diet closer to that practiced by non-celiac persons.

CONSENT FOR PUBLICATION

Not applicable.

CONFLICT OF INTEREST

The author confirms this chapter contents have no conflict of interest.

ACKNOWLEDGEMENTS

Declared none.

REFERENCES

Bascuñán, K.A., Vespa, M.C., Araya, M. (2017). Celiac disease: understanding the gluten-free diet. *Eur. J. Nutr., 56*(2), 449-459.
[http://dx.doi.org/10.1007/s00394-016-1238-5] [PMID: 27334430]

Cappello, M., Morreale, G.C., Licata, A. (2016). Elderly onset celiac disease: A narrative review. *Clin. Med. Insights Gastroenterol., 9*, 41-49.
[http://dx.doi.org/10.4137/CGast.S38454] [PMID: 27486350]

Ciacci, C., Ciclitira, P., Hadjivassiliou, M., Kaukinen, K., Ludvigsson, J.F., McGough, N., Sanders, D.S., Woodward, J., Leonard, J.N., Swift, G.L. (2015). The gluten-free diet and its current application in coeliac disease and dermatitis herpetiformis. *United European Gastroenterol. J., 3*(2), 121-135.
[http://dx.doi.org/10.1177/2050640614559263] [PMID: 25922672]

Czaja-Bulsa, G., Bulsa, M. (2018). Adherence to gluten-free diet in children with celiac disease. *Nutrients, 10*(10)E1424
[http://dx.doi.org/10.3390/nu10101424] [PMID: 30287732]

Edwards, E. A., Lumsden, J., Rivas, C., Steed, L., Edwards, L. A., Thiyagarajan, A., Walton, R. T. (2016). Gamification for health promotion: systematic review of behaviour change techniques in smartphone apps 6(10), e012447.

Guiraldes, E., Gutierrez, C. (1988). Coeliac disease and Holy Communion. *Lancet, 1*(8575-6), 57.
[http://dx.doi.org/10.1016/S0140-6736(88)91036-7]

Gujral, N., Freeman, H. J., Thomson, A. B. R. (2012). Celiac disease : Prevalence , diagnosis , pathogenesis and treatment 18(42), 6036-6059.

Heredia-Sandoval, N.G., Valencia-Tapia, M.Y., Calderón de la Barca, A.M., Islas-Rubio, A.R. (2016). Microbial Proteases in Baked Goods: Modification of Gluten and Effects on Immunogenicity and Product

Quality. *Foods,* 5(3), 59.
[http://dx.doi.org/10.3390/foods5030059] [PMID: 28231153]

Institute of Medicine Committee on Health L. (2004). Health Literacy: A Prescription to End Confusion. Washington (DC): National Academies Press (US) Copyright 2004 by the National Academy of Sciences. All rights reserved.

Jouanin, A., Boyd, L., Visser, R.G.F., Smulders, M.J.M. (2018). Development of Wheat With Hypoimmunogenic Gluten Obstructed by the Gene Editing Policy in Europe. *Front. Plant Sci., 9,* 1523-1523.
[http://dx.doi.org/10.3389/fpls.2018.01523] [PMID: 30405661]

Ka, H., Na, B., Genet, N., Ea, S., Genet, P., Ea, S. (2014). New Epidemiology of Celiac Disease, 59(July), 7-9.

Kang, J. Y., Kang, A. H. Y., Green, A., Gwee, K. A., Ho, K. Y. (2013). *Alimentary Pharmacology and Therapeutics Systematic review : worldwide variation in the frequency of coeliac disease and changes over time.*
[http://dx.doi.org/doi.org/10.1111/apt.12373]

Levin-Zamir, D., Bertschi, I. (2018). Media health literacy, eHealth literacy, and the role of the social environment in context. *Int. J. Environ. Res. Public Health, 15*(8), 1643.
[http://dx.doi.org/10.3390/ijerph15081643] [PMID: 30081465]

Morreale, F., Agnoli, C., Roncoroni, L., Sieri, S., Lombardo, V., Mazzeo, T., Elli, L., Bardella, M.T., Agostoni, C., Doneda, L., Scricciolo, A., Brighenti, F., Pellegrini, N. (2018). Are the dietary habits of treated individuals with celiac disease adherent to a Mediterranean diet? *Nutr. Metab. Cardiovasc. Dis., 28*(11), 1148-1154.
[http://dx.doi.org/10.1016/j.numecd.2018.06.021] [PMID: 30143412]

Muhammad, H., Reeves, S., Ishaq, S., Mayberry, J., Jeanes, Y.M. (2017). Adherence to a gluten free diet is associated with receiving gluten free foods on prescription and understanding food labelling. *Nutrients, 9*(7), E705.
[http://dx.doi.org/10.3390/nu9070705] [PMID: 28684693]

Newnham, E.D., Shepherd, S.J., Strauss, B.J., Hosking, P., Gibson, P.R. (2016). Adherence to the gluten-free diet can achieve the therapeutic goals in almost all patients with coeliac disease: A 5-year longitudinal study from diagnosis. *J. Gastroenterol. Hepatol., 31*(2), 342-349.
[http://dx.doi.org/10.1111/jgh.13060] [PMID: 26212198]

Park, K., Harris, M., Khavari, N., Khosla, C. (2014). Rationale for Using Social Media to Collect Patient-Reported Outcomes in Patients with Celiac Disease. *J. Gastrointest. Dig. Syst., 4*(1), 166.
[http://dx.doi.org/10.4172/2161-069x.1000166] [PMID: 25392743]

Rewers, M. (2005). Epidemiology of Celiac Disease: What Are the Prevalence, Incidence, and Progression of Celiac Disease?, 47-51.
[http://dx.doi.org/10.1053/j.gastro.2005.02.030]

Silvester, J.A., Weiten, D., Graff, L.A., Walker, J.R., Duerksen, D.R. (2016). Is it gluten-free? Relationship between self-reported gluten-free diet adherence and knowledge of gluten content of foods. *Nutrition, 32*(7-8), 777-783.
[http://dx.doi.org/10.1016/j.nut.2016.01.021] [PMID: 27131408]

Stein, R.A., Katz, D.E. (2017). Celiac Disease. *Foodborne Diseases.* Academic Press.
[http://dx.doi.org/10.1016/B978-0-12-385007-2.00024-3]

Therrien, A., Kelly, C. (2018). *Celiac Disease: The Right Clinical Information, Right where It's Needed.* BMJ Best Practice.

Vaquero, L., Rodríguez-Martín, L., León, F., Jorquera, F., Vivas, S. (2018). New coeliac disease treatments and their complications. *Gastroenterol. Hepatol., 41*(3), 191-204. [English Edition].
[http://dx.doi.org/10.1016/j.gastrohep.2017.12.002] [PMID: 29422237]

Ventola, C. L. (2014). Mobile devices and apps for health care professionals: uses and benefits. *P & T : J Formul Manag* 39(5), 356-364.

Vici, G., Belli, L., Biondi, M., Polzonetti, V. (2016). Gluten free diet and nutrient deficiencies: A review. *Clin. Nutr.,* 35(6), 1236-1241.
[http://dx.doi.org/10.1016/j.clnu.2016.05.002] [PMID: 27211234]

Zarkadas, M., Dubois, S., MacIsaac, K., Cantin, I., Rashid, M., Roberts, K. C., Pulido, O. M. (2013). Living with coeliac disease and a gluten-free diet. *Can Pers* 26(1), 10-23.
[http://dx.doi.org/10.1111/j.1365-277X.2012.01288.x]

CHAPTER 8

Animal-Assisted Therapy and Developmental Disorders

Gladys Malafaia[1,*], **Sofia Santos**[2] and **Pedro Morato**[1]

[1] *Faculdade de Motricidade Humana, Universidade de Lisboa, Lisboa, Portugal*

[2] *Faculdade de Motricidade Humana, UIDEF – Instituto da Educação, Universidade de Lisboa, Lisboa, Portugal*

Abstract: For the last few years, neurosciences has been focusing its research on analysing the structures and processes behind Animal-Assisted Therapies (AAT) and their effects on persons with neurodevelopmental disorders. The aim of this study is to present an overview of the main evidence-based effects of AAT in the promotion of skills, health-related issues, and well-being of persons with neurodevelopmental disorders. For this matter, the main theories of AAT effects will be approached. In conclusion, animal-human interaction characteristics and how this relationship may compensate deficits and promote functional competences will be described.

Keywords: Animal-assisted therapy, Attention deficit and hyperactivity disorder, Autism, Developmental disorders, Health, Learning disability, Well-being.

INTRODUCTION

Animal-Assisted Therapy (AAT) conceptualization is due to Boris Levinson, in the sixties, within his experience in assessing the effects of using animals in therapeutic processes (Bachi & Parish-Plass, 2016). Levinson called his dog Jingles a "pet partner" (Levinson, 1964). The use of animals as promotors of human development has been consistently reported through time (Fine, 2015), although not all interventions are therapeutic and the animal could not be considered as the therapist although may assume the role of mediator or facilitator (Bachi & Parish-Plass, 2016). The integration of an animal in therapy seems to facilitate a therapeutic alliance, as one of the key aspects in this dynamic (Wesley, Minatrea & Watson, 2009), intensifying the interaction between physiological and psychological (Odendaal, 2000).

The interest in AAT application with persons with developmental disorders has

---

[*] **Corresponding author Gladys Malafaia:** Faculdade de Motricidade Humana, Universidade de Lisboa, Lisboa, Portugal; E-mail: gladysmalafaia@hotmail.com

been increasing for last two decades (Hart & Yamamoto, 2015), due to its relevance and it is being used with different subgroups across lifespan, from children and adolescents (Balchi, 2013; Balluerka, Muela, Amiano, & Caldentey, 2015) to older people (Filan & Llewellyn-Jones, 2006), with and without developmental (O'Haire, 2012), or psychiatric disorders (Nathans-Barel, Feldman, Berger, Modai, & Silver, 2005), war Veterans (Yount, Ritchie, St. Laurent, Chumley, & Olmert, 2013) and prisoners (Bachi, 2013), and within distinct settings such as classrooms (Gee, Church, & Altobelli, 2015; Smith & Dale, 2016), hospitals (Braun, Stangler, Narveson, & Pettingell, 2009; Giuliania & Jacquemettaza, 2017; Johnson, Meadows, Haubner, & Sevedge, 2003; Marcus, *et al.*, 2012), home (Heade, Fu, & Zheng, 2008), or rehabilitative context (Muñoz, *et al.*, 2015).

This animal incorporation in therapeutic processes seems to be beneficial for persons with supports needs and positive evidences are reported in literature especially in cases of anxiety, stress, depression, challenging behaviors, attention deficits, ability to be involved in tasks, motivation, learning disabilities, motor coordination, social, and communications disorders (Beetz, Julius, Turner, & Kotrschal, 2012; Hart & Yamamoto, 2015; Herzog, 2017; Julius, Beetz, Kotrschal, Turner, & Uvnäs-Moberg, 2013; Odendaal & Meintjes, 2003; Seal, Robinson, Kelly, & Williams, 2013).

As this article is focused on the relation between AAT and groups with developmental disorders, its definitions should be clear. Developmental disorders involve a set of changes that occur during the central nervous system' development that usually are expressed in early years and characterized by limitations on critical developmental acquisitions at several levels: sensorimotor, cognitive, socioemotional, adaptive, behaviour, and communication, which affect human functioning (American Association Psychiatric [APA], 2013). Examples of developmental disorders include intellectual and developmental disability, communication disorders, autism spectrum disorder, attention-deficit/hyperactivity disorder (ADHD), specific learning disabilities, motor disability, among others (APA, 2013).

Animal-Assisted Therapies

Terminology in AAT has varied tremendously across times, and terms are often used interchangeably, according to each therapeutic process aim (recreational, therapeutic, *etc.* - Kruger & Serpell, 2010). Therefore, some of the most used terms will be briefly defined.

Animal-Assisted Activities (AAA) are informal/casual interactions between person-animal, with rigid criteria or goals, used for motivational, educational, and recreational purposes (Pet Partners, 2012). The same references add that there are no therapeutic aim or previous established goals, as well as no planning or evaluation, and are traditionally facilitated by individuals without training in health, education, or social services. Kruger & Serpell (2010) reported that AAA are directed towards the improvement of quality of life by motivational, recreational, and educational components, through the recruitment of an animal with specific characteristics.

Human-Animal Interaction (HAI) can be defined as a dynamic and mutual interchange between human beings and animals, influenced by components, essential for both health and well-being, within environmental demands (American Veterinary Medical Association [AVMA], 2018). According to this association, this bond includes and is influenced by physical, emotional, and psychological interactions between humans, animals, and the environment.

AAT or Animal-Assisted Interventions (AAI), which is the most used term, encompasses pedagogical and psychological interventions with therapeutic aims and goals, adapted to each person or groups of individuals that include the active participation of an animal within structures activities performed by habilitated health professionals (Pet Partners, 2012). This is a controlled and documented process, with results and progress monitoring. The main goal of AAT/AAI is to improve motor, cognitive, socioemotional, and behavioral functions and animals play an essential role in all therapeutic processes (Pet Partners, 2012).

The *European Society for Animal-Assisted The*rapy (ESAAT, 2011), based on International Classification of Functioning, Health, and Disability (ICF, World Health Organization [WHO], 2001), defines AAT as pedagogical and psychological interventions that aim to promote health, prevent, and rehabilitate symptoms, using trained animals, trying to match support needs with supports provision, according to high ethical standards. It bases its approach in the interaction of three elements: client(s), animal, and therapist.

The main goals of AAT (ESAAT, 2011) are the promotion of well-being and quality of life through personal competences stimulation for real and active social participation, across the lifespan. AAT seeks the cognitive, motor, and socioemotional rehabilitation and its maintenance through activities and treatment interventions led by trained professionals in the health field: psychotherapist, psychology, education, *etc*. The specific goals are bases on the support's needs, strengths, and weaknesses identification, as well in resources available (ESAAT, 2011). In all these processes of AAT, some legal requisites that support interventions should be considered: animals' protection and physical and psychological well-being should be ensured, hygiene standards to prevent zoonosis (infectious diseases transmitted by animals to humans), insurance and responsibility documentation in order, therapist qualification, animal training, therapeutic environment analyses (for a better interaction between animal-human), and even the cost of all processes – including veterinarian care and adequate food (ESAAT, 2004).

Theory of Animal Assisted Therapy

Animals are strong positive mediators in cognitive, socio-emotional, and learning domains (Beetz, 2017), with positive effects in neurobiological components, such as stress reduction (Julius, Beetz, Kotrschal, Turner & Uvnäs, 2013). However, only in the last two decades, scientific research found positive evidence between animal companion and personal well-being (Wells, 2009). Further, there is increasing interest in human-animal interaction' mechanisms (*e.g.*: attachment theories, biophilia, and social support hypothesis), which are interrelated in a complex process.

From the neurophysiologic point of view, the right hemisphere is responsible for emotional regulation and mental health with direct consequences in personal and social behavior adjustment (Geist, 2011). A person that is not able to self-control increases the probability of physical, emotional, and behavioral stress, which is influenced by the attachment quality in the neuronal activation that allows the representation of the experience. In this sense, AAT may act as facilitators of healthy and affective experiences, through more secure relations between humans and animals, allowing a better adaptation to environmental demands (Geist, 2011; Zilcha-Mno, Mikulincer, & Shaver, 2011).

According to the attachment theory, there is a biological predisposition, either in humans and animals, to seek emotional and physical connections with and in certain living systems (Sable, 2013). If this connection is positive, then healthy and positive self-esteem will be developed, and if the connection is negative, it may lead to insecure and uncertainty states (Geist, 2011; Kovács, Bulucz, Kis, & Simon, 2006). The animal, in the AAT context, will assume the mediator role, improving the contact with the person (Bacchi, 2013a) and replacing other bonding figures (Mallon, 1992).

Socio-emotional support hypothesis (Uchino, 2006) is related with group interaction, and with behaviors and psychological attitudes that promote physical activities, touch and physical contact, self-control, putting cardiovascular, neuroendocrine and immunologic systems in action. Once more, the animal assumes an important role in securing social relations, especially with persons with disorganized or insecure attachments processes (Beetz *et al.*, 2012a), which physiological indicators are low levels of cortisol and cardiovascular responses, contributing for stress regulation (Odendaal & Meintjes, 2003).

The biophilia hypothesis, like stated before, is directly related with the natural predisposition to seek connections with nature and other forms of life and its stimulation properties (Beck & Katcher, 2003), as well with psychological (endorphins production) well-being effects and physiological effects in (active and positive) relationships established between human and nature (Kellert & Wilson 1993, cit. in Ulrich, 1993). AAT seek the comforting touch and attachment evolution in the presence of companion animals, and the ability to establish successful interpersonal relations (Levinson, 1965).

Cognitive theory is based on the continuous and reciprocal interaction between the cognitive system, environmental demands, and human behaviour (Kruger & Serpell, 2010). Again, attachment is crucial for the creation of positive or negative feelings that influence action (Geist, 2011), self-efficacy, personal fulfilment, and personal condition (Fine, 2010). The significance given to events will limit the behavioral response and so the positive relation with the animal may lead to healthy attachments and a positive self-concept (Geist, 2011). That is why animals were rapidly used in therapy, to allow cause-effect conscience (Fine, 2015).

Additionally, all these elements may influence positive results of these interaction such as Anthropomorphism (*i.e.*: attribution of human traits, emotions, or intentions to animals), allowing to stay focused on experience, rather than verbal communication, due to the motivation and distraction brought by the animal in the therapeutic process (Wohlfarth, Mutschler, Beetz e Schleider, 2014). Through the AAT's therapeutic process, the approach type, individual preferences, the adequate animal, and the context in which the animal is expected to function according to treatment goals, benefits anticipation, and proposal viability should be considered (Sockalingam *et al.*, 2008). The recognition of these therapeutic process effects, although still scarce, points out the long-term effects in several domains, and so main benefits will be briefly described.

Effects

The positive consequences of humans and animals' interactions are well documented in the literature, with individuals of all ages and with physical and psychological conditions. The most consensual and reported benefits are related to attention, social attention and behaviour, humour, interpersonal relations, stress indicators (cortisol, heart rate, and blood pressure), fear and anxiety, physical and mental health, and cardiovascular diseases (Beetz, Uvnäs-Moberg, Julius, & Kotrschal, 2012b). Animals can have a tremendous impact on neurobiological/physiological domains, learning, and social processes and so the next section will present them.

Neurobiological

The knowledge of neurobiological mechanisms and its consequences at physiological level is fundamental to understand the importance of the animal integration in therapeutic processes with children with developmental disorders, such as autism spectrum disorder, for a significant reduction of stress reactions in social contexts, impacting the anxiety levels as well the confidence in communicating with their peers (Beetz & Bales, 2016). Scientific evidence supports AAT as a neuro-hormonal regulator process (oxytocin and cortisol), directly connected with anxiety processes (Cole, Gawlinski, Steers, & Kotlerman, 2007; Odendaal & Meintjes, 2003). These authors observed that sensorial stimulation, by interacting with dogs, led to the brain and circulatory system' endorphins release with an impact in physical pain reduction and a higher sense of well-being. The neurotransmitter oxytocin, associated with physical pleasure, was also released (Beetz, 2017; Odendaal & Meintjes, 2003).

The influence of AAT (Marcus *et al.*, 2012) showed then animal mediation results in increase of endorphins production, with a major impact in well-being feelings, improving the immunologic response, and activating the parasympathetic system, responsible for the deaccelerating of heart beatings, decrease of blood pressure and respiratory rhythm, increase of periphery skin temperature, which are all actions that allow the human body to recognize the proper answer for relaxation and calm conditions. With adults, the visits of dogs allowed a significant pain reduction and more advantage responses to treatment.

Charnetski, Riggers, & Brennan (2004) analyzed the impact of using animals (dogs) in immunological function specifically in immunoglobulin A (IgA) antibody production, whose main function is to protect against pathogens (viruses or bacteria's) present in body secretions and inhibit the inflammatory effect of others immunoglobulins produced by mucous. Fifty-five participants, randomly distributed for three groups, were evaluated in three different moments: firstly, they pet real dogs, then pet toy-dogs, and finally, they sat comfortably. The analysis showed the significant increase of IgA levels in pre and post real dog pet situations, pointing out the important role that this contact may have in fighting infections.

Physiological

Evidence in animal mediation in physiological human processes has also been reported in research, with positive relations within the health domain: less need for doctor appointments, decrease of medication, and improvement in general physical health (Heade *et al.*, 2008). Following the positive results towards the impact of AAT in neurotransmitters, some authors analyzed AAT impact in pain reduction which affect, significantly, its inherent physiological mechanisms, matching the animal interaction with children in a therapeutic environment with oral medicines or pain killers (Braun *et al.*, 2009; Johnson *et al.*, 2003; Marcus *et al.*, 2012). Results showed a decrease of cortisol levels, with an active role in blood pressure and heart rate, due to its relation with adrenalin, which have an important role in the way how humans face stressing situations (Viau, *et al.*, 2010). Similar results were found by Sobo, Brenda, & Kassity-Krich (2006) who assessed (pre and post) 25 children hospitalized who were submitted to previous surgery and were in pain, found a significant decrease of pain after each AAT session.

Psychological

The integration of animals in therapeutic processes may help to potentiate the cognitive development, relaxation ability, self-esteem, and events acceptance, orientation towards reality, confidence, stress and anxiety reduction, learning, loneliness decrease, positive affection, loneliness decrease, empathy, concentration, and intrinsic motivation, among others (Beetz, 2017). Children with challenging behaviors are at risk for most severe emotional disorders in adolescence, which may potentiate serious psychopathologies in adult life. So, positive and effective interventions as early as possible are fundamental for emotional development (Ewing, MacDonald, Taylor, & Bower, 2007). The authors point out the ability of animals to obtain trust and attention, especially from teenagers and adolescents. Another important element for behavior organization, and that usually is compromised in persons with challenging behavior, is the empathy need. Animals are able to shorten the distance between person and mediator, due to its role as activities-partner, favouring social competences acquisition, like consideration and respect for others, being able to transfer this empathy to human beings (Praglin & Nebbe, 2014).

Scientific evidences of the positive impact of a (therapeutic) animal presence are reported in literature in cognitive performance, such as objects classification and categorization or motor skills, in pre-school children with and without developmental disorders (Gee *et al.*, 2015; Wohlfarth, Mutschler, Beetz, Kreuser, & Korsten-Reck, 2013; Wohlfarth *et al.*, 2014). Using a dog as a therapeutic mediator seems to have beneficial effects on implicit motivation. This was observed by Wohlfarth and colleagues (2013) who assessed 13 children with obesity in the performance of physical tasks. The improvements were also verified at reading level namely at words and punctuation signals recognition, as well the use of such signals at the end of paragraphs. Anxiety (Van Steensel, Boögel, & Perrin, 2011) and depression (Souter & Miller, 2007) levels were also analyzed and results seem to corroborate the AAT effectiveness with both subgroups.

AAT seems to benefit perceived stress. Wu, Niedra, Pendergast, & McCrindle (2002) analyzed the effects of therapeutic dogs 10-20 minutes' visits to children, and results showed a stress decrease and the improvement of humour either from children, as their parents. Hyoung-Joon & Chung-Hui (2012) study results suggest that 12 sessions of 60 minutes' AAT, using companion animals, have a positive significant influence in the self-esteem of adolescents suffering from depression and low self-esteem due to scholar violence. Results seem to indicate the need for less time for such interventions, for emotional stability and more stable effects through time. Taking care of an animal offers many opportunities to promote executive functioning: animals are not self-sufficient and the responsibility of taking care of them (feeding, exercising, rest, *etc*.) will guide and structure children activities (Lino, Kelly, & Diamond, 2016)

Learning

The learning process demands several components such as attention, motivation, concentration, among others, but also stress and fear absence (Blakemore & Frith, 2005). For the past years, AAT scientific evidence tends to indicate its benefits in several domains (Friesen, 2010), including scholar learning processes (*e.g.*: in sciences, mathematics, health, social studies, *etc*.).

Children with learning disabilities show limitations in keeping attention and interest in challenging tasks, with consequences at anxiety, stress, agitation, challenging behaviors, among others(Giuliania & Jacquemettaza, 2017). The neurobiological stimulation potential of dogs seems to decrease the stress and anxiety levels of these children, refocusing the attention for the animal interaction and promoting participation in tasks with others with joy being a source of motivation and safety. Hoffmann and colleagues (2009) found identical results especially, and Gee, Church & Altobelli (2015) specified these important effects at cognitive tasks and problem solving. Even in scholar settings, the interaction between animals and students favours the development of motor skills, through game creation and tasks that demand fine and gross motor skills (Chandler, 2001). Therapy dogs can also be used as a catalyser to promote and motivate children to be more actively engaged in physical activities (Wohlfarth, Mutschler, Beetz, Kreuser, & Korsten-reck, 2013).

Sometimes, schools are the only place where children have the opportunity to engage in physical activity, although is not enough. The effectiveness of using a dog as a therapy-mediator in the promotion of physical activity engagement of 12 participants, between 8 and 12 years, with obesity (Body Mass Index in 90-97 percentile) was measured (Wohlfarth *et al.*, 2013). All participants received an accelerometer to measure activity. In the first session, the dog was near two children and had to do some agility exercises and children were asked to be faster than the dog. In the next session, the dog was not there and the same type of previously described exercises had to be performed. Results showed a significant reduction of passivity when the dog was present. Further, children presented a considerable distance difference as well walking time difference, if in the dog presence (*vs.* without the dog presence). The authors suggested that the dog's presence acts as an enjoyable stimulus for physical activity engagement.

Social

Under an evolutionary perspective, humans and animals share social and cerebral structures and mechanisms, which give different species the ability to socialize (Beetz, Julius, Turner, & Kotrschal, 2012; Julius, Beetz, Kotrschal, Turner, & Uvnäs-Moberg, 2013). The interaction with animals influences social relations between humans including respect, confidence, empathy, and positive humour, and as before, acts as a social catalyser promoting interpersonal positive relations and socialization (Prothmann, Bienert, & Ettrich, 2006). Children with autism spectrum disorder have significant limitations in communication and social interaction, and embracing or talking to animals or therapists could promote more positive social behaviors (Sams, Fortney, & Willenbring, 2006). Similar results were found by Rusu (2016) with a child with educational supports needs and a diagnosis of intellectual disability and attention deficit and hyperactivity disorder.

ANIMAL-ASSISTED THERAPY IN NEURODEVELOPMENTAL DISORDERS

Based on the literature review, it is possible to find some evidences about the interaction with an animal within the AAT context. The dog is frequently considered as children (with and without disability) "special friends", offering unique social support (Nicholas & Collis, 2000). The dog spontaneous enthusiasm for social interaction may act as a stimulus to increase children's social behaviours (Giuliania & Jacquemettaza, 2017; Prothmann *et al.*, 2006).

The presence of the dog leads to more positive behaviors such as smiles and pleasant physical contact, as well as the decrease of stereotypes and repetitive behaviors by children with autism spectrum disorder (Funahashi, Gruebler, Aoki, Kadone, & Suzuki, 2014). AAT can be a process to reinforce concentration, improve sensorial stimulus receptivity and communication with others, aiming a better quality of life as a result of the improved psychological well-being, social development and motor proficiency (Siewertsen, French, & Teramoto, 2015). The authors added a decrease in physiological reactions to anxiety and stress. AAT also have positive results in motivation and executive functioning of children with attention-deficit and hyperactivity disorder, expressed in a better social ability to establish interpersonal relations (Schuck, Emmerson, Fine & Lakes, 2015). Animals are primary motivators of positive emotional responses, acting as catalyzers to learning (Fine, 2015). Similar findings were found with children with intellectual disability (Vivaldin & De Oliveira, 2011) and motor disability.

CONCLUDING REMARKS

Generally speaking, AAT (being the dog one of the main/primary incorporated animal) seems to have positive consequences in the independent functioning, social participation, and quality of life persons with neurodevelopmental disorders (Funahashi *et al.*, 2014; Schuck *et al.*, 2015; Siewertsen *et al.*, 2015; Srinivasan, Caravagnino, & Bhat, 2018; Vivaldin & de Oliveira, 2011). Attention and motivation have a major impact on learning processes, and animals can promote positive emotional answers in these areas through multiple experiences and optimizing the effects of the intervention (Fine, 2015). The development of verbal and non-verbal communication and social relations (Rusu, 2016), based on an effective attachment between person and animal (Roley *et al.*, 2015), and the improvement of motor proficiency (McPhillips, Finlay, Bejerol, & Hanley, 2018; Srinivasan *et al.*, 2018) are some of the domains that might benefit by the incorporation of animals in therapeutic contexts (Ajzenman, Standeven, & Shurtleff, 2013).

In spite of the recent interest in research about AAT and the potential role played by the incorporation of an animal in therapeutic settings, more scientific studies about the AAT efficacy and how these eventual changes can be rigorously measured are recommended. Some of the main critics to research in the area are the study length's limitations, the differences between samples, the lack of outcome results generalization, and the need to have a valid comprehension about the scope of animal therapeutic involvement.

Evidence-based knowledge will allow future and more adjusted decisions about the strategies and protocols to be put into action in the rehabilitation field, with groups with different support needs and in distinct areas (health, social...), *i.e.*, best practices. Ethical considerations either for humans as for animals should be considered.

CONSENT FOR PUBLICATION

Not applicable.

CONFLICT OF INTEREST

The author confirms that this chapter contents have no conflict of interest.

ACKNOWLEDGEMENTS

Declared none.

REFERENCES

Ajzenman, H.F., Standeven, J.W., Shurtleff, T.L. (2013). Effect of hippotherapy on motor control, adaptive behaviors, and participation in children with autism spectrum disorder: a pilot study. *Am. J. Occup. Ther., 67*(6), 653-663.
[http://dx.doi.org/10.5014/ajot.2013.008383] [PMID: 24195899]

American Veterinary Medical Association. (2013). *American Psychiatric Association: Diagnostic and Statistical Manual of Mental Disorders.* (5th ed.). Arlington, VA: American Psychiatric Association.

American Veterinary Medical Association. (2018). *The Human-Animal Interaction and Human-Animal Bond.* Research made at 18 November and retrieved from https://www.avma.org/Pages/home.aspx

Bachi, K. (2013). Equine-facilitated prison-based programs within the context of prison-based animal programs: State of the science review. *J. Offender Rehabil., 52*, 46-74.
[http://dx.doi.org/10.1080/10509674.2012.734371]

Bachi, K., Parish-Plass, N. (2017). Animal-assisted psychotherapy: A unique relational therapy for children and adolescents. *Clin. Child Psychol. Psychiatry, 22*(1), 3-8.
[http://dx.doi.org/10.1177/1359104516672549] [PMID: 27742758]

Balluerka, N., Muela, A., Amiano, N., Caldentey, M.A. (2015). Promoting psychosocial adaptation of youths in residential care through animal-assisted psychotherapy. *Child Abuse Negl., 50*, 193-205.
[http://dx.doi.org/10.1016/j.chiabu.2015.09.004] [PMID: 26443670]

Beetz, A. (2017). Theories and possible processes of action in animal assisted interventions. *Appl. Dev. Sci., 21*, 139-149.
[http://dx.doi.org/10.1080/10888691.2016.1262263]

Beetz, A., Bales, K. (2016). Affiliation in human-animal interaction. In: Freund, L. S., McCune, S., Esposito, L., Gee, N. R., McCardle, P., (Eds.), *The Social Neuroscience of Human–Animal Interaction.* USA: American Psychological Association.
[http://dx.doi.org/10.1037/14856-007]

Beetz, A., Julius, H., Turner, D., Kotrschal, K. (2012). Effects of social support by a dog on stress modulation in male children with insecure attachment. *Front. Psychol., 3*(352), 352.
[http://dx.doi.org/10.3389/fpsyg.2012.00352] [PMID: 23162482]

Beetz, A., Uvnäs-Moberg, K., Julius, H., Kotrschal, K. (2012). Effects of social support by a dog on stress modulation in male children with insecure attachment. *Front. Psychol, 3*(352), 1-9.
[http://dx.doi.org/10.3389/fpsyg.2012.00352]

Blakemore, S-J., Frith, U. (2005). *The Learning Brain: Lessons for Education.* Wiley-Blackwell.

Braun, C., Stangler, T., Narveson, J., Pettingell, S. (2009). Animal-assisted therapy as a pain relief intervention for children. *Complement. Ther. Clin. Pract., 15*(2), 105-109.
[http://dx.doi.org/10.1016/j.ctcp.2009.02.008] [PMID: 19341990]

Charnetski, C.J., Riggers, S., Brennan, F.X. (2004). Effect of petting a dog on immune system function. *Psychol. Rep., 95*(3 Pt 2), 1087-1091.
[http://dx.doi.org/10.2466/pr0.95.3f.1087-1091] [PMID: 15762389]

Cole, K.M., Gawlinski, A., Steers, N., Kotlerman, J. (2007). Animal-assisted therapy in patients hospitalized with heart failure. *Am. J. Crit. Care, 16*(6), 575-585.
[PMID: 17962502]

European Society for Animal Assisted Therapy. (2011). *Definition "Animal Assisted Therapy.* retrieved at 10th October 2018 from http://goo.gl/Rzaikz

Ewing, C., MacDonald, P., Taylor, M., Bower, M. (2007). Equine-Facilitated Learning for Youths with Severe Emotional Disorders: A Quantitative and Qualitative Study. *Child Youth Care Forum, 36*, 59-72.
[http://dx.doi.org/10.1007/s10566-006-9031-x]

Filan, S.L., Llewellyn-Jones, R.H. (2006). Animal-assisted therapy for dementia: a review of the literature. *Int. Psychogeriatr., 18*(4), 597-611.
[http://dx.doi.org/10.1017/S1041610206003322] [PMID: 16640796]

Fine, A. (2015). *Handbook on Animal Assisted Therapy. Theoretical Foundations and Guidelines for Practice.* (4th ed.). San Diego, USA: Elsevier Inc..

Friesen, L. (2010). Exploring animal-assisted programs with children in school and therapeutic contexts. *Early Child. Educ. J., 37*, 261-267.
[http://dx.doi.org/10.1007/s10643-009-0349-5]

Funahashi, A., Gruebler, A., Aoki, T., Kadone, H., Suzuki, K. (2014). Brief report: the smiles of a child with autism spectrum disorder during an animal-assisted activity may facilitate social positive behaviors--quantitative analysis with smile-detecting interface. *J. Autism Dev. Disord., 44*(3), 685-693.
[http://dx.doi.org/10.1007/s10803-013-1898-4] [PMID: 23893100]

Gee, N., Church, M., Altobelli, C. (2015). Preschoolers make fewer errors on an object categorization task in the presence of a dog. *Antrozoös, 223-230.
[http://dx.doi.org/10.2752/175303710X12750451258896]

Geist, T. (2011). Conceptual framework for animal assisted therapy. *Child Adolesc. Soc. Work J., 28*, 243-256.
[http://dx.doi.org/10.1007/s10560-011-0231-3]

Giuliania, F., Jacquemettaza, M. (2017). Animal-assisted therapy used for anxiety disorders in patients with learning disabilities: An observational study. *Eur. J. Integr. Med., 14*, 13-19.
[http://dx.doi.org/10.1016/j.eujim.2017.08.004]

Hart, L. & Yamamoto, M. (2015). Recruiting Psychosocial Health Effects of Animals for Families and Communities: Transition to Practice. In Fine, A., (Ed). *Handbook on Animal-Assisted Therapy.* Foundations and Guidelines for practice (pp. 53-72). Academic Press.
[http://dx.doi.org/10.1016/B978-0-12-801292-5.00006-7]

Heade, B., Fu, N., Zheng, R. (2008). Pet dogs benefit owners' health: A "Natural Experiment" in China. *ERIC, 87*, 481-493.
[http://dx.doi.org/10.1007/s11205-007-9142-2]

Herzog, H. (2017). Why Do People Tink Animals Make Good Terapists? *Animal Studies Repository,* 1-5.

Hoffmann, A., Lee, A., Wertenauer, F., Ricken, R., Jansen, J., Gallinat, J., Lang, U.E. (2009). Dog-assisted interventions significantly reduces anxiety in hospitalized patients with major depression. *Eur. J. Integr. Med., 1*, 145-148.
[http://dx.doi.org/10.1016/j.eujim.2009.08.002]

Hyoung-Joon, P., Chung-Hui, K. (2012). The Effects of an Animal-Assisted Therapy (AAT) Program on Depression and Self-esteem of Adolescents as Victims of School Violence. *Kor. J. Vet. Serv., 35*, 56-68.
[http://dx.doi.org/10.7853/kjvs.2012.35.4.327]

Johnson, R., Meadows, R., Haubner, J., Sevedge, K. (2003). Human-animal interaction. A complementary/alternative medical (CAM) intervention for cancer patients. *Am. Behav. Sci., 47*, 55-69.
[http://dx.doi.org/10.1177/0002764203255213]

Julius, H., Beetz, A., Kotrschal, K., Turner, D., Uvnäs-Moberg, K. (2013). *Attachment to Pets - An Integrative View of Human-Animal Relationships with Implications for Therapeutic Practice.* New York: Hogrefe.

Julius, H., Beetz, A., Kotrschal, K., Turner, D., Uvnäs-Moberg, K. (2013). *Attachment to Pet: An Integrative View of Human–Animal Relationships with Implications for Therapeutic Practice.* Hogrefe.

Kovács, Z., Bulucz, J., Kis, R., Simon, L. (2006). An exploratory study of the effects of animal-assisted therapy on nonverbal comunication in three schizophrenic patients. *Anthrozoos, 4*, 353-364.
[http://dx.doi.org/10.2752/089279306785415475]

Kruger, K., Serpell, J. (2010). Animal-assisted interventions in mental health: definitions and theoretical foundations. *Handbook on Animal-Assisted Therapy Theoretical Foundations and Guidelines for Practice.* (3rd ed., pp. 33-48). USA: Elsevier.
[http://dx.doi.org/10.1016/B978-0-12-381453-1.10003-0]

Levinson, B. (1965). Pet psychotherapy: use of household pets in the treatment of behavior disorder in childhood. *VI International Congress of Psychotherapy, in London,* 695-698.England: Southern Universities Press.
[http://dx.doi.org/10.2466/pr0.1965.17.3.695]

Lino, D., Kelly, M., Diamond, A. (2016). Human-Animal Interaction and the Development of Executive Functions. In: Freund, L. S., McCune, S., Esposito, L., Gee, N. R., McCardle, P., (Eds.), *The Social Neuroscience of Human-Animal Interaction.* (pp. 51-72). Washinton, DC: American Psychological Association.

Mallon, G. (1992). Utilization of animals as therapeutic adjuncts with children and youth: a review of the literature. *Child Youth Care Forum, 2*, 53-67. [New York: Human Sciences Press Inc.].
[http://dx.doi.org/10.1007/BF00757348]

Marcus, D.A., Bernstein, C.D., Constantin, J.M., Kunkel, F.A., Breuer, P., Hanlon, R.B. (2012). Animal-assisted therapy at an outpatient pain management clinic. *Pain Med., 13*(1), 45-57.
[http://dx.doi.org/10.1111/j.1526-4637.2011.01294.x] [PMID: 22233395]

McPhillips, M., Finlay, J., Bejerot, S., Hanley, M. (2014). Motor deficits in children with autism spectrum disorder: a cross-syndrome study. *Autism Res., 7*(6), 664-676.
[http://dx.doi.org/10.1002/aur.1408] [PMID: 25258309]

Muñoz, L., Bocanegra, M., Valero, A., Atín, A., Varela, D., Ferriero, G. (2015). Intervenciones asistidas por animales en neurorehabilitación: una revisión de la literatura más reciente. *Neurologia, 30*, 1-7.
[http://dx.doi.org/10.1016/j.nrl.2013.01.012]

McNicholas, J., Collis, G.M. (2000). Dogs as catalysts for social interactions: robustness of the effect. *Br. J. Psychol., 91*(Pt 1), 61-70.
[http://dx.doi.org/10.1348/000712600161673] [PMID: 10717771]

Odendaal, J.S., Meintjes, R.A. (2003). Neurophysiological correlates of affiliative behaviour between humans and dogs. *Vet. J., 165*(3), 296-301.
[http://dx.doi.org/10.1016/S1090-0233(02)00237-X] [PMID: 12672376]

O'Haire, M.E. (2013). Animal-assisted intervention for autism spectrum disorder: a systematic literature review. *J. Autism Dev. Disord., 43*(7), 1606-1622.
[http://dx.doi.org/10.1007/s10803-012-1707-5] [PMID: 23124442]

(2012). *Pet Partners - Touchin lives through human-animal interactions.* retrieved from Animal-assisted therapy: http://www.petpartners.org/page.aspx?pid=320

Praglin, L., Nebbe, L. (2014). Introduction to Animal- and Nature-Assisted Therapies: A Service-Learning Model for Rural Social Work. *Contemp. Rural Soc. Work, 6*, 146-157.

Prothmann, A., Albrecht, K., Dietrich, S., Hornfeck, U., Stieber, S., Ettrich, C. (2005). Analysis of child-dog play behavior in child psychiatry. *Anthrozoos, 18*, 43-58.
[http://dx.doi.org/10.2752/089279305785594261]

Prothmann, A., Bienert, M., Ettrich, C. (2006). Dogs in Child Psychotherapy: Effects on State of Mind. *Anthrozoos: Multidiscipli. J. Interact. People Anim., 19*, 265-277.

Roley, S.S., Mailloux, Z., Parham, L.D., Schaaf, R.C., Lane, C.J., Cermak, S. (2015). Sensory integration and praxis patterns in children with autism. *Am. J. Occup. Ther., 69*(1)6901220010 [http://dx.doi.org/10.5014/ajot.2015.012476] [PMID: 25553746]

Rusu, A. (2016). *An Interdisciplinary Approach of Animal Assisted Therapy for the Special Needs Children. ERD 2016: Education, Reflection, Development.* (4th ed., p. 9). UK: Future Academy.

Sams, M.J., Fortney, E.V., Willenbring, S. (2006). Occupational therapy incorporating animals for children with autism: A pilot investigation. *Am. J. Occup. Ther., 60*(3), 268-274.
[http://dx.doi.org/10.5014/ajot.60.3.268] [PMID: 16776394]

Schuck, S.E., Emmerson, N.A., Fine, A.H., Lakes, K.D. (2015). Canine-assisted therapy for children with ADHD: preliminary findings from the positive assertive cooperative kids study. *J. Atten. Disord., 19*(2), 125-137.
[http://dx.doi.org/10.1177/1087054713502080] [PMID: 24062278]

Seal, A., Robinson, G., Kelly, A., Williams, J. (2013). *Children with Neurodevelopmental Disabilities. The Essential Guide to Assessment and Management.* London: Mac Keith Press.

Siewertsen, C.M., French, E.D., Teramoto, M. (2015). Autism spectrum disorder and pet therapy. *Adv. Mind Body Med., 29*(2), 22-25.
[PMID: 25831431]

Smith, B., Dale, A. (2016). Integrating animals in the classroom: The attitudes and experiences of Australian school teachers toward animal-assisted interventions for children with Autism. *Pet Behav. Sci., 1*, 13-22.
[http://dx.doi.org/10.21071/pbs.v0i1.3994]

Sobo, E.J., Eng, B., Kassity-Krich, N. (2006). Canine visitation (pet) therapy: pilot data on decreases in child pain perception. *J. Holist. Nurs., 24*(1), 51-57.
[http://dx.doi.org/10.1177/0898010105280112] [PMID: 16449747]

Sockalingam, S., Li, M., Krishnadev, U., Hanson, K., Balaban, K., Pacione, L.R., Bhalerao, S. (2008). Use of animal-assisted therapy in the rehabilitation of an assault victim with a concurrent mood disorder. *Issues Ment. Health Nurs., 29*(1), 73-84.
[http://dx.doi.org/10.1080/01612840701748847] [PMID: 18214780]

Souter, M., Miller, M. (2007). Do animal-assisted activities effectively treat depression? A meta-analysis. *Anthrozoos, 20*, 167-180.
[http://dx.doi.org/10.2752/175303707X207954]

Srinivasan, S.M., Cavagnino, D.T., Bhat, A.N. (2018). Effects of equine therapy on individuals with autism spectrum disorder: A systematic review. *Rev. J. Autism Dev. Disord, 5*(2), 156-175.
[http://dx.doi.org/10.1007/s40489-018-0130-z] [PMID: 30319932]

Ulrich, R. (1993). Biophilia, Biophobia and Natural Landscapes. *The Biophilia Hypothesis.* (pp. 73-137). USA: Island Press.

van Steensel, F.J., Bögels, S.M., Perrin, S. (2011). Anxiety disorders in children and adolescents with autistic spectrum disorders: a meta-analysis. *Clin. Child Fam. Psychol. Rev., 14*(3), 302-317.
[http://dx.doi.org/10.1007/s10567-011-0097-0] [PMID: 21735077]

Viau, R., Arsenault-Lapierre, G., Fecteau, S., Champagne, N., Walker, C-D., Lupien, S. (2010). Effect of service dogs on salivary cortisol secretion in autistic children. *Psychoneuroendocrinology, 35*(8), 1187-1193.
[http://dx.doi.org/10.1016/j.psyneuen.2010.02.004] [PMID: 20189722]

Vivaldin, V., De Oliveira, V. (2011). Terapia assistida por animais em reabilitação clínica de pessoas com deficiência intelectual *31*, 527-544.

Wells, D. (2009). The effects of animal on human health and well-being. *J. Soc. Issues, 65*, 523-543.
[http://dx.doi.org/10.1111/j.1540-4560.2009.01612.x]

Wohlfarth, R., Mutschler, B., Beetz, A., Kreuser, F., Korsten-Reck, U. (2013). Dogs motivate obese children for physical activity: key elements of a motivational theory of animal-assisted interventions. *Front. Psychol., 4*, 796.
[http://dx.doi.org/10.3389/fpsyg.2013.00796] [PMID: 24194726]

Wohlfarth, R., Mutschler, B., Beetz, A., Schleider, K. (2014). An investigation into the efficacy of therapy dogs on reading performance in 6-7 year old children. *Hum. Anim. Interact. Bull., 2*, 60-73.

World Health Organization. (2001). *International Classification of Functioning, Disability and Health.* Geneva: WHO Library.

Wu, A.S., Niedra, R., Pendergast, L., McCrindle, B.W. (2002). Acceptability and impact of pet visitation on a pediatric cardiology inpatient unit. *J. Pediatr. Nurs., 17*(5), 354-362.
[http://dx.doi.org/10.1053/jpdn.2002.127173] [PMID: 12395303]

Yount, R., Ritchie, E., St. Laurent, M., Chumley, P., Olmert, M. (2013). The role of service dog training in the treatment of combat-related PTSD. *Psychiatr. Ann., 43*, 292-295.

Zilcha-Mano, S., Mikulincer, M., Shaver, P.R. (2011). Pet in the therapy room: an attachment perspective on Animal-Assisted Therapy. *Attach. Hum. Dev., 13*(6), 541-561.
[http://dx.doi.org/10.1080/14616734.2011.608987] [PMID: 22011099]

CHAPTER 9

Physical Activity Practice Determinants for People with Motor Disabilities: Inequities in Access and Physical Activity Engagement

Bárbara Almeida[1], Sofia Santos[2,*], Fernando Gomes[3] and **Adilson Marques[4]**

[1] *Faculdade de Motricidade Humana, Universidade de Lisboa, Portugal*

[2] *Faculdade de Motricidade Humana, UIDEF – Instituto da Educação, Universidade de Lisboa, Portugal*

[3] *SpertLab, Faculdade de Motricidade Humana, Universidade de Lisboa, Portugal*

[4] *CIPER, Faculdade de Motricidade Humana, Universidade de Lisboa, Faculdade de Motricidade Humana, Estrada da Costa, 1499-002 Cruz Quebrada, Portugal*

Abstract: Even with extensive documentation on the health benefits of physical activity (PA), a part of the population does not practice enough PA to have these benefits, especially people with disabilities. People with motor disabilities tend to be less engaged in PA than their peers, even with the positive outcomes on bodily, social, functional and emotional changes promoted by PA. Therefore, the identification and knowledge of PA's determinants, either as facilitators or barriers, for people with motor disabilities seems logical and essential. The goal of this chapter is to review the literature about these determinants and examine possible future paths. This information can contribute to conceptual changes and new interventions and policies that increase the levels of PA practice in this population subgroup and, consequently, further advance their social inclusion.

Keywords: Barriers, Determinants, Facilitators, Motor disabilities, Physical activity.

INTRODUCTION

The benefits of physical activity (PA) are well documented (Hardman & Stensel, 2009), namely in the maintenance of health and physical fitness (World Health Organization, 2016) for people with or without disabilities (Murphy, Carbone & Council on Children with Disabilities, 2008). In general, PA regular practice contributes to the reduction of musculoskeletal and cardiovascular diseases, obesity (Marques, Sarmento, Martins & Nunes, 2015b), increased personal and

* **Corresponding author Sofia Santos:** Faculdade de Motricidade Humana, UIDEF – Instituto de Educação, Universidade de Lisboa, Portugal; Tel: +351214149243; E-mail: sofiasantos@fmh.ulisboa.pt

social autonomy, community integration, self-esteem (Biddle & Asare, 2011), stress and anxiety reduction (Hogan, Catalino, Mata & Fredrickson, 2015; Murphy ., 2008), *etc*. PA is a predictor of better health, regardless of other factors such as age, sex, socioeconomic status, body mass index, smoking, and educational level (WHO, 2007).

Despite its health benefits, a considerable part of the population does not practice PA as recommended (European Commission, 2018; Marques *et al*., 2015b; Marques, Martins, Peralta, Catunda & Nunes, 2016) and in recent decades, there have been major changes in lifestyle, characterized by increased levels of sedentarism (Ng & Popkin, 2012). Physical inactivity and sedentary behaviors represent a health problem, with particular emphasis on subgroups with low socioeconomic status and people with some type of limitation or disability (Bauman *et al*., 2012).

PA is a behavior that varies in form and context and can be considered a biocultural process, therefore, its approach requires the understanding of its determinants (Rimmer, Riley, Wang, Rauworth, & Jurkowski, 2004). Habits and lifestyles are not always the result of entirely free, conscious and autonomous choices, being influenced by external, environmental, social, cultural, and economic pressures and constraints (*e.g.*: gender, age, physical fitness, environmental, social, cultural and psychological factors), and thereby needing a multidisciplinary approach (Seabra, Mendonça, Thomis, Anjos & Maia, 2008).

The lack of involvement of people with disabilities in PA and/or theirs physical inactivity is a current fact (Badia, Orgaz, Verdugo & Ullan, 2013; Solish, Perry & Minnes, 2010), with a tendency towards sedentarism. Factors that may influence or discourage PA practice in this population subgroup are diverse. People with intellectual disabilities identify determinants linked to support and the scarcity of information about PA programs, with proper follow-up; people with visual impairment tend to refer to determinants linked to family support and to the professionals skills (Rimmer & Rowland, 2008); and people with motor disabilities tend to identify more environmental determinants such as accessibility of facilities or means of transportation and travel, as well as factors associated with bodily functionality (Rimmer *et al*., 2004).

Physical limitations, associated with increased therapeutic needs, poor economic status, psychological impairment or lack of accessibility, contribute to a less healthy lifestyle (Bedell *et al*., 2013). Therefore, PA engagement has a positive impact on the life of a person with motor disabilities. Motor disability is characterized as any physical alteration in the human body, resulting from some orthopaedic, neurological or congenital malformation problems (Mauerberg de

Castro, 2005), with developmental impairments and repercussions on performing varied motor tasks. In addition, there is a greater tendency for the development of chronic diseases, such as diabetes, hypertension and obesity (Anderson & Heyne, 2010; Riley, Rimmer, Wang & Schiller, 2008).

The search for the practice of PA by the person with motor disability, as well as any other type of disability, can contribute to the rehabilitation process, as a means of testing possibilities, preventing secondary diseases and promoting the total integration of the individual in the society (Zabriskie, Lundberg & Groff, 2005). The authors emphasize the importance of participation in recreational activities, particularly highlighting the well-being and the development of the feeling of competence (King *et al.*, 2003; Safania & Mokhtari, 2012), social recognition with social networking and positive impact of interaction with typical peers (Hassan, Dowling, McConkey, & Menke, 2012; Wilhite & Shank, 2009). The prevention of functional decline (Murphy *et al.*, 2008) and the maintenance of functional independence are also worth mentioning (Rimmer *et al.*, 2004).

Therefore, it is important to understand why people with motor disabilities have lower levels of PA, when it could bring, in addition to the common benefits, increased mobility, functionality and autonomy, body strengthening in the face of physical limitation and positive emotional reinforcement, interaction and social inclusion (Barclay, MacDonald, Lentin & Bourke-Taylor, 2016; Marques, Maldonado, Peralta & Santos, 2015a). People with motor disability tend to have higher values of body mass index, lower levels of flexibility, strength, endurance and speed (Hands & Larkin, 2006), and regular practice of PA is associated with proven benefits (Rimmer & Rowland, 2008; United States Department of Health and Human Services, 2018).

The low accessibility and adherence to PA should be seen as one of the public health concerns (Eck *et al.*, 2008; WHO, 2016). A healthy lifestyle should be understood as a key point in reducing the risk factors for the health of people with disabilities thus highlighting the importance of PA in this field (WHO, 2016). The prevalence of inactivity, characteristic of people with disabilities, is related to medical, psychological, social or involvement barriers, *etc.* (Martin, 2013).

Currently, there are still few studies that address the determinants of the PA practice in people with motor deficits (Rimmer *et al.*, 2004; Seabra *et al.*, 2008) and the consequent non-participation in PA on a regular basis (Roberts, Cavill, Hancock & Rutter, 2013), in school, social or recreational context. The identification and understanding of these determinants leads to the discovery of the mechanisms through which the behavior is controlled or modified. The knowledge is used to establish, among others, intervention programs. This group of determinants is multifactorial, involving personal and social factors (Belley-Ranger *et al.*, 2016b), which influence the quality and quantity of participation of all people (Belley-Ranger, Duquette, Carbonneau & Roult, 2016a), with and without a disability. The next section will address the set of determinants that influence sports and PA.

Determinants

Crawford & Godbey (1987) made the first attempt to categorize the determinants, grouping them into intrapersonal, interpersonal, and structural determinants; later, they were categorized as intrinsic, environmental, and communicational (Smith, Cheung, Bauman, Zehle & McLean, 2005). Personal and involvement determinants (Jaarsma, Dijkstra, Blécourt, Geertzen & Dekker, 2014) are currently recognized. In this chapter, the determinants of the practice of PA will be presented in four different groups: sociodemographic, psychological, involvement and social.

Sociodemographic Determinants

Demographic factors, such as age or gender, influence PA practice, which is significantly lower in adulthood, with the decline in practice with age (Craggs, Corder, van Sluijs & Griffin, 2011; Matos *et al.*, 2012), in spite of decline-evidence based in young people (Hills, King & Armstrong, 2007). Some longitudinal studies suggest that sedentary children and adolescents tend to maintain this negative behavior throughout their lives, which may put them at risk of greater morbidity (Bauman, 2004). Even with compulsory school participation (*e.g.*: physical education classes), children and adolescents with motor disability practice significantly less PA than their typical peers (Maher, Williamns, Olds & Lane, 2007; Rimmer & Rowland, 2008). The prevalence of greater activity among males is verified (Matos *et al.*, 2012), with females being more inactive.

In the context of the socioeconomic status, the research is not very consensual regarding the existence of its relationship with the practice of PA (Sallis, Prochaska & Taylor, 2000; Van der Horst, Paw, Twisk & Van Mechelen, 2007). Evidence suggests that when there is an association between these factors, there is a trend towards a growing practice of PA for people with better socioeconomic status, despite lack of analysis in the field of motor disability (Maher *et al.*, 2007). Only 3% of individuals with motor disability practice PA regularly, although 50% of these individuals show interest in practicing (Perrier, Shirazipour & Latimer-Cheung, 2015).

Carlon, Taylor, Dodd & Shields (2013) found lower rates of participation in PA by young people with cerebral palsy, with 13 to 53% lower values compared with their typical peers, and 30% below PA practice guidelines. In the Netherlands, children with severe motor impairment showed significantly lower values in PA, with a prevalence of a higher level of overweight and obesity (Neter *et al.*, 2011). In general, a low socioeconomic status can be considered a risk in adopting a more inactive lifestyle (WHO, 2007). Furthermore, the lack of financial support for the practice of PA, both in terms of maintenance and on-site trips, has been pointed out as a limitation to a more active and healthier lifestyle (Slater & Tiggemann, 2010).

Other demographic characteristics, such as ethnicity and cultural patterns, have also been investigated, but the information is still inconsistent (Malina & Little, 2008): some studies seem to indicate that Caucasian individuals tend to be physically more active than individuals of other ethnicities (Sallis *et al.*, 2000). However, the number of studies indicating that there is no relationship between these variables and the PA practice are also significant (Van der Horst *et al.*, 2007).

Physical and intellectual limitations may also determine the level and practice of PA. These limitations, associated with poor self-esteem, inadequate surrounding space, or lack of conditions for practice restricted physical activity (Mulligan *et al.*, 2012). This may reflect a lack of information about their real possibilities (Serona, Arruda & Greguol, 2015).

The fundamental motor skills (*e.g.*: locomotion, manipulation, stability, among others) are considered important for the development of more specific movements, and are all required in PA engagement; if compromised, they become a barrier, not only for the limitations themselves but also for all their consequences on physical, cognitive and social development. Motor proficiency during childhood and the practice of PA in adolescence are significant and influence the perception of competence, increasing subsequent commitment to this practice (Barnett, Morgan, van Beurden & Beard, 2008).

Pain is another determinant which is considered important for the PA practice, particularly associated with specific disabilities, such as motor disability. This factor can be considered a barrier when it restricts practice, or as a facilitator, when PA engagement prevents or reduces pain (Bragaru *et al.*, 2013).

Psychological Determinants

Within psychological and emotional areas, there are other types of determinants, such as intention and the motivation which are positively associated with PA engagement (Van der Horst *et al.*, 2007). Motivation, an intrinsic determination to achieve a goal, is crucial to the performance of any behavior and, therefore also in self-promotion of well-being and health through PA. On the other hand, the intention is a motivational component, being the intention to be active or not determinant in the involvement in the practice of PA. Both rely heavily on capacity and competence perception and on other factors, including involvement factors (Sallis *et al.*, 2000).

The body image, or awareness of a person from an affective and emotional perspective, as it is felt and experienced by the individual (Gürsel & Koruç, 2011), is another determinant reported by the literature. It is something complex, involving perceptions, attitudes and beliefs about the body itself - therefore it is subjective, but has a strong social determination (Rodrigues, 2005). This image is influenced by several factors, such as the image that is socially accepted as normal or ideal. When referring to people with disabilities, this perception changes, since this condition refers directly to the body (structures and functions) limitation, which can lead to a disbelief in its capacities and competencies and to a lower level of self-esteem (Bauman *et al.*, 2012). Body image has been related to lower levels of PA in females, although it is transversal to gender and age (Biddle & Asare, 2011).

As previously mentioned, self-esteem is linked with body image (Craggs *et al.*, 2011), which is also associated with ability and competence' perception. Competency perception measures the degree of personal effectiveness relative to one's abilities to perform specific behaviors. This perception may indicate the tendency to be physically active and to promote physical and psychological well-being (Bauman *et al.*, 2012). The perception of one's own abilities and competencies contributes, in a general way, to greater self-esteem and motivation that, in turn, is reflected in successful PA practice (Marques *et al.*, 2009).

People with disabilities have lower self-esteem and perception of skills compared to their peers (Pijl & Frostad, 2010). Perception of efficiency means trusting your actions. . It is distinguished from the perception of capacity and competence, since this is the personal perception of what the person can and cannot do; and self-efficiency refers to an intrinsic force for action, where independently of its perception, the person believes he will be able to act (Bauman *et al.*, 2012). According to the authors, the efficiency perception theory indicates that the confidence in performing a behavior is strongly related to the ability to perform this same behavior and, therefore, is also linked to the performance. Thus, individuals with high self-efficacy are more likely to act and persevere in the face of new challenges, also applying to the involvement in the practice of PA.

The information and value attributed to health and the understanding of the benefits of PA also influence positively the way in which this practice is evolved

(Sallis *et al.*, 2000), although some inconclusive results (Craggs *et al.*, 2011). In general, the perception of benefits in PA has positive associations with this practice thus facilitating and promoting action. The perceived benefits are varied and depend on each person. Children and adolescents with more positive health perceptions are more likely to practice PA regularly, recognizing their benefits (Rowe, Raedeke, Wiersma & Mahar, 2007). On the other hand, when the perception of barriers overlaps, the practice of PA is compromised. The false idea that PA does not bring relevant benefits to people with disabilities is a significant deterrent to their practice (Rimmer *et al.*, 2004). Therefore, is important to promote the acquisition of this information, assuming it as a key part of this whole question.

Although considered to be a determining factor, amusement does not have a significantly positive relationship with PA engagement (Biddle & Asare, 2011). Nevertheless, it is considered important as pleasure and success in PA engagement, motivate its continuity. It is suggested that amusement may be more important for females. Associated with fun is participation in leisure PA. In this context, participation rates are quite low among people with disabilities, with an estimated 56% of these people not performing physical leisure activities (Cardinal, Kosma, & McCubbin, 2004; Ginis, Nigg & Noreau, 2013).

Finally, previous PA behavior appears to play a relevant role in future practice, and therefore the mechanisms underlying this association need to be better understood. It is observed that there is a continuity in the practice of physical activity throughout these periods (Bauman *et al.*, 2012). In addition, habits also influence AF practice, including eating habits (Sallis *et al.*, 2000; Van der Horst *et al.*, 2007). For people with or without disabilities, a healthy diet is positively related to physical activity.

Involvement Determinants

The determinants of involvement are associated with external characteristics of both the physical and social surroundings: infrastructure conditions, transportation, among others, are examples of factors that influence the PA engagement (Sallis *et al.*, 2000). All personal, physical, and behavioral intentions for activity change according to will, social, psychological, and biological reinforcement.

Accessibility is a key and decisive point in the practice of PA by people with motor disabilities. The first issues associated are the infrastructure conditions, the physical conditions of the surrounding space, and the existence of suitable equipment (Craike, Symons & Zimmermann, 2009). However, accessibility is also reflected in having trained professionals for monitoring people with disabilities' in PA engagement; means of transport suitable for on-the-spot travel; or even questions of interrelated nature, such as the perception of negative attitudes on the part of others present in the space. All of this, in parallel with the personal determinants that, per se, already have a great influence on the decision making (Craike *et al.*, 2009; Humbert *et al.*, 2008).

Architectural construction and infrastructures are aspects that stand out in a first approach. People with motor disabilities have a variety of limitations, often physical ones, such as reduced mobility, which require adapted conditions. However, the focus should not be on people with disabilities, but rather on environmental adaptation . This issue is relevant for people with disabilities, including the promotion of an active lifestyle and the PA engagement, which are greatly influenced by environmental characteristics (Ferreira & Najar, 2005). Appropriate transport is another concern in this matter (Slater & Tiggemann, 2010).

Social Determinants

Although strongly determinant in the decision to PA practice, most physical barriers can be overcome when there is adequate support from both the family and peers as well as from significant adults and skilled professionals. All the beliefs and attitudes of family members, friends and people with disabilities themselves can act as barriers or facilitators for the PA engagement (Ferreira & Najar, 2005).

The influence of the family in PA engagement focuses on the modeling of interests and abilities, enhancing their continuity in the future, being significantly greater throughout childhood and adolescencent stages in which lifestyles are established, but lengthening throughout life, especially among people with disabilities, since they are often dependent on their support (Sérgio, 2005).

The importance of peers seems to strengthen with age. The relationship between the degree of disability, self-perception and interaction with typical peers, can lead to different attitudes and behaviors towards society (Sérgio, 2005). If, on the one hand, peers can be a support in the integration of a new school, helping to minimize academic difficulties, on the other hand, there are also discriminatory attitudes of avoidance and rejection when the adult is not present (Malheiro, 2005). The preference of the peers for other kinds of activities, rather than PA, influences inactivity or previous negative experiences with PA being identified as a barrier (Coleman, Cox & Roker, 2008; Craike *et al.*, 2009; Slater & Tiggemann, 2010). Inactive relatives or lack of encouragement are examples of barriers to the practice of PA (Coleman *et al.*, 2008; Slater & Tiggemann, 2010; Rimmer & Rowland, 2008). However, the support provided by family and friends can be positive and serve as a facilitator, when PA engagement is encouraged.

In a different scope are the social and legal support, *i.e.*, the available opportunities for participation in PA and their adequate organization. Although significant progress has been made, disability is still seen as a challenge to the public health system, especially because of the lack of knowledge, by health professionals, about the particularities of disabilities and how to deal with them (Rimmer, Chen, McCubbin, Drum & Peterson, 2010). Besides being a fundamental right, PA is seen as a unique opportunity for the maintenance of health and autonomy, thus favouring the development of educational values and social inclusion (Lollar, 2002).

The lack of available PA programs or knowledge about those already available, coupled with disinformation by professionals, means that the person with a disability has few opportunities to become active thus further deteriorating their quality of life (Lollar, 2002). Unfortunately, there are few opportunities for these people to successfully engage in PA programs. Disability does not mean poor health and does not justify a lesser investment in promoting good habits to ensure positive health. There are scarce projects in basic health care for people with disabilities, and existing programs for the general population present difficulties for the inclusion of people with disabilities (Othero & Dalmaso, 2009). It is important to emphasize that often the limitation of people with disabilities is not in the "organic gravity of their condition" or in the functional behaviors, but rather in complex social processes that influence social inequalities among citizens. The identification of these factors and the establishment of an individual profile provides useful information for the development of intervention programs that enhance PA engagement by people with motor disabilities (Bloemen *et al.*, 2014).

It should be noted that lack of PA programs is widespread both in schools and in the community (Azzarito & Hill, 2013; Craike *et al.*, 2009), which combined with accessibility barriers, monetary issues or lack of specialized and qualified professional support, among others, will limit PA engagement of persons with motor disabilities. It is important to intervene in this issue and invest in the creation of public, community and inclusive programs, identifying the perceptions of people with disabilities about the benefits and barriers to PA and integrating in the design of these actions. It should be noted that the few supervised programs available may often not meet the interests and needs of people with disabilities (Rimmer *et al.*, 2010). The existence of more opportunities for participation in PA is a matter of concern, and the lack of programs contribute to the rate of sedentarism, with all the consequences associated with it. In addition, estimates indicate that physically more active populations, with healthier lifestyles, contribute to the reduction of costs related to public health (Pitanga, 2002).

Finally, it is important to mention the role of the school in promoting the practice of PA. The school is the main institution capable of influencing people to adopt an active lifestyle through inclusive and quality Physical Education programs (WHO, 2010; Pate *et al.*, 2006). Since there are few AF practice opportunities outside the context of school, educational work, especially with family and other caregivers, can lead to improvements in behaviors and the adoption of a healthier lifestyle (Hinckson, Dickinson, Water, Sands & Penman, 2013). Studies show that the opportunity to practice PA in school is fundamental for children and adolescents with disabilities (Valis & Gonzalez, 2016) because it enhances the continuity of this practice in the long term.

The school context seems to be one of the means, par excellence, for the acquisition of healthy living habits by all students, with and without disabilities (De, Small & Baur, 2008), despite the many constraints - inaccessibility of structures and stigmatization (Belley-Ranger *et al.*, 2016a) with which students with disabilities are faced (Roult, Carbonneau, Chan, Belley-Ranger & Duquette, 2014), resulting in reduced opportunities for curricular and extracurricular practice at school or even in the surrounding community (Carbonneau & Roult, 2013).

For many students with disabilities, physical education classes at school are one of the few opportunities to experience varied motor experiences, being a socially relevant territory. It is in this context that many children and adolescents have the only opportunity to have access to quality physical activity experiences, adapted to their possibilities, giving them the opportunity to be valued in the world (Lehnhard, Manta & Palma, 2012). Unfortunately, it seems still far from fully including all students. Although many children with disabilities even have access to regular school, in many cases, they are dismissed from Physical Education classes, usually because of the teacher's insecurity (Corbin, 2002).

CONCLUDING REMARKS

Although the health benefits of PA have been widely documented, a part of the population does not practice enough PA to have these benefits, especially people with disabilities. People with motor disabilities tend to be less engaged in PA than their typical peers. Therefore, the identification and knowledge of the PA's determinants for this population's subgroup are essential, as well as the reflection on possible future paths to improve and promote those who are positive and facilitators of the engagement in PA.

Four different groups of PA determinants have been identified: sociodemographic, psychological, and social involvement, such as facilitators or as barriers, with an impact on PA engagement. It is relevant to focus on the facilitators and strategies to overcome barriers, keeping in mind its inter-influence. One strong facilitator can suppress other determinants acting as barriers. This information can contribute to conceptual changes and new interventions and policies that increase the levels of PA practice and, consequently, further advance their full social inclusion.

CONSENT FOR PUBLICATION

Not applicable.

CONFLICT OF INTEREST

The author confirms that this chapter contents have no conflict of interest.

ACKNOWLEDGEMENTS

Declared none.

REFERENCES

Anderson, L.S., Heyne, L.A. (2010). Physical activity for children and adults with disabilities: An issue of "amplified" importance. *Disabil. Health J., 3*(2), 71-73.
[http://dx.doi.org/10.1016/j.dhjo.2009.11.004] [PMID: 21122770]

Azzarito, L., Hill, J. (2013). Girls looking for a 'second home': Bodies, difference and places of inclusion. *Phys. Educ. Sport Pedagogy, 18*(4), 351-375.
[http://dx.doi.org/10.1080/17408989.2012.666792]

Badia, M., Orgaz, M.B., Verdugo, M.Á., Ullán, A.M. (2013). Patterns and determinants of leisure participation of youth and adults with developmental disabilities. *J. Intellect. Disabil. Res., 57*(4), 319-332.
[http://dx.doi.org/10.1111/j.1365-2788.2012.01539.x] [PMID: 22404152]

Barclay, L., McDonald, R., Lentin, P., Bourke-Taylor, H. (2016). Facilitators and barriers to social and community participation following spinal cord injury. *Aust. Occup. Ther. J., 63*(1), 19-28.
[http://dx.doi.org/10.1111/1440-1630.12241] [PMID: 26530379]

Barnett, L.M., Morgan, P.J., van Beurden, E., Beard, J.R. (2008). Perceived sports competence mediates the relationship between childhood motor skill proficiency and adolescent physical activity and fitness: A longitudinal assessment. *Int. J. Behav. Nutr. Phys. Act., 5*, 40.
[http://dx.doi.org/10.1186/1479-5868-5-40] [PMID: 18687148]

Bauman, A.E. (2004). Updating the evidence that physical activity is good for health: An epidemiological review 2000-2003. *J. Sci. Med. Sport, 7*(1) (Suppl.), 6-19.
[http://dx.doi.org/10.1016/S1440-2440(04)80273-1] [PMID: 15214597]

Bauman, A.E., Reis, R.S., Sallis, J.F., Wells, J.C., Loos, R.J., Martin, B.W. (2012). Correlates of physical activity: Why are some people physically active and others not? *Lancet, 380*(9838), 258-271.
[http://dx.doi.org/10.1016/S0140-6736(12)60735-1] [PMID: 22818938]

Bedell, G., Coster, W., Law, M., Liljenquist, K., Kao, Y.C., Teplicky, R., Anaby, D., Khetani, M.A. (2013). Community participation, supports, and barriers of school-age children with and without disabilities. *Arch. Phys. Med. Rehabil., 94*(2), 315-323.
[http://dx.doi.org/10.1016/j.apmr.2012.09.024] [PMID: 23044364]

Belley-Ranger, E., Carbonneau, H., Roult, R., Brunet, I., Duquette, M-M., Nauroy, E. (2016). Determinants

of participation in sport and physical activity for students with disabilities according to teachers and school-based practitioners specialized in recreational and competitive physical activity. *Sport Sci. Rev., 25*(3-4), 135-158. b
[http://dx.doi.org/10.1515/ssr-2016-0008]

Belley-Ranger, E., Duquette, M., Carbonneau, H., Roult, R. (2016). Interactions with peers in physical and sporting activities among students with functional limitations in Quebec. *World Leis.*
[http://dx.doi.org/10.1080/16078055.2015.1107619]

Biddle, S.J., Asare, M. (2011). Physical activity and mental health in children and adolescents: A review of reviews. *Br. J. Sports Med., 45*(11), 886-895.
[http://dx.doi.org/10.1136/bjsports-2011-090185] [PMID: 21807669]

Bloemen, M., Backx, F., Takken, T., Wittink, H., Benner, J., Mollema, J., Groot, J. (2014). Factors associated with physical activity in children and adolescents with a physical disability: A systematic review. *Dev. Med. Child Neurol., 15*(1), 1-12.
[http://dx.doi.org/10.1111/dmcn.12624] [PMID: 25403649]

Bragaru, M., van Wilgen, C.P., Geertzen, J.H., Ruijs, S.G., Dijkstra, P.U., Dekker, R. (2013). Barriers and facilitators of participation in sports: A qualitative study on Dutch individuals with lower limb amputation. *PLoS One, 8*(3), e59881.
[http://dx.doi.org/10.1371/journal.pone.0059881] [PMID: 23533655]

Carbonneau, H., Roult, R. (2013). *Rapport sur l'étude des facteurs facilitant l'adoption de saines habitudes de vie et la pratique d'activités physiques et sportives par les jeunes ayant une limitation fonctionnelle.* Département d'Études en loisir, culture et tourisme UQTR – Défi Sportif.

Cardinal, B.J., Kosma, M., McCubbin, J.A. (2004). Factors influencing the exercise behavior of adults with physical disabilities. *Med. Sci. Sports Exerc., 36*(5), 868-875.
[http://dx.doi.org/10.1249/01.MSS.0000126568.63402.22] [PMID: 15126723]

Carlon, S.L., Taylor, N.F., Dodd, K.J., Shields, N. (2013). Differences in habitual physical activity levels of young people with cerebral palsy and their typically developing peers: A systematic review. *Disabil. Rehabil., 35*(8), 647-655.
[http://dx.doi.org/10.3109/09638288.2012.715721] [PMID: 23072296]

Coleman, L., Cox, L., Roker, D. (2008). Girls and young women's participation in physical activity: Psychological and social influences. *Health Educ. Res., 23*(4), 633-647.
[http://dx.doi.org/10.1093/her/cym040] [PMID: 17897930]

Corbin, C. (2002). Physical education as an agent of change. *Quest, 54*(3), 182-195.
[http://dx.doi.org/10.1080/00336297.2002.10491773]

Craike, M., Symons, C., Zimmermann, J. (2009). Why do young women drop out of sport and physical activity? A social ecological approach. *Ann. Leis. Res., 12*(2), 148-172.
[http://dx.doi.org/10.1080/11745398.2009.9686816]

Craggs, C., Corder, K., van Sluijs, E.M., Griffin, S.J. (2011). Determinants of change in physical activity in children and adolescents: A systematic review. *Am. J. Prev. Med., 40*(6), 645-658.
[http://dx.doi.org/10.1016/j.amepre.2011.02.025] [PMID: 21565658]

Crawford, D., Godbey, G. (1987). Reconceptualizing Barriers to Family Leisure. *Leis. Sci., 9*(2), 119-127.
[http://dx.doi.org/10.1080/01490408709512151]

De, S., Small, J., Baur, L.A. (2008). Overweight and obesity among children with developmental disabilities. *J. Intellect. Dev. Disabil., 33*(1), 43-47.
[http://dx.doi.org/10.1080/13668250701875137] [PMID: 18300166]

van Eck, M., Dallmeijer, A.J., Beckerman, H., van den Hoven, P.A., Voorman, J.M., Becher, J.G. (2008). Physical activity level and related factors in adolescents with cerebral palsy. *Pediatr. Exerc. Sci., 20*(1), 95-106.
[http://dx.doi.org/10.1123/pes.20.1.95] [PMID: 18364538]

European Commission. (2018). *Sport and physical activity. Special Eurobarometer 472..* Brussels: European Commission, Directorate-General for Education and Culture and co-ordinated by Directorate-General for Communication.

Ferreira, M., Najar, A. (2005). Programas e campanhas de promoção da atividade física *Ciência & Saúde Coletiva, 10*, 207-219.
[http://dx.doi.org/10.1590/S1413-81232005000500022]

Ginis, K.A., Nigg, C.R., Smith, A.L. (2013). Peer-delivered physical activity interventions: An overlooked opportunity for physical activity promotion. *Transl. Behav. Med., 3*(4), 434-443.
[http://dx.doi.org/10.1007/s13142-013-0215-2] [PMID: 24294332]

Gürsel, F., Koruç, Z. (2011). The influence of physical activity on body image in people with and without acquired mobility disability. *Acta Universitatis Palackianae Olomucensis, 41*(4), 29-35.
[http://dx.doi.org/10.5507/ag.2011.023]

Hands, B., Larkin, D. (2006). Physical fitness differences in children with and without motor learning difficulties. *Eur. J. Spec. Needs Educ., 21*(4), 447-456.
[http://dx.doi.org/10.1080/08856250600956410]

Hassan, D., Dowling, S., McConkey, R., Menke, S. (2012). The inclusion of people with intellectual disabilities in team sports: Lessons from the youth unified sports porogramme of Special Olympics. *Sport Soc., 15*(9), 1275-1290.
[http://dx.doi.org/10.1080/17430437.2012.695348]

Hardman, A., Stensel, D. (2009). *Physical activity and health. The evidence explaine*d. Oxford: Routledge.Hills, Hinckson, E., Dickinson, A., Water, T., Sands, M. & Penman, L. (2013). Physical activity, dietary habits and overall health in overweight and obese children and youth with intellectual disability or autism. *Res. Dev. Disabil., 34*(4), 1170-1178.
[http://dx.doi.org/10.1016/j.ridd.2012.12.006]

Hogan, C.L., Catalino, L.I., Mata, J., Fredrickson, B.L. (2015). Beyond emotional benefits: Physical activity and sedentary behaviour affect psychosocial resources through emotions. *Psychol. Health, 30*(3), 354-369.
[http://dx.doi.org/10.1080/08870446.2014.973410] [PMID: 25307453]

Humbert, M.L., Chad, K.E., Spink, K.S., Muhajarine, N., Anderson, K.D., Bruner, M.W., Girolami, T.M., Odnokon, P., Gryba, C.R. (2006). Factors that influence physical activity participation among high- and low-SES youth. *Qual. Health Res., 16*(4), 467-483.
[http://dx.doi.org/10.1177/1049732305286051] [PMID: 16513991]

Jaarsma, E.A., Dijkstra, P.U., de Blécourt, A.C., Geertzen, J.H., Dekker, R. (2015). Barriers and facilitators of sports in children with physical disabilities: A mixed-method study. *Disabil. Rehabil., 37*(18), 1617-1623.
[http://dx.doi.org/10.3109/09638288.2014.972587] [PMID: 25347764]

King, G., Law, M., Hanna, S., King, S., Hurley, P., Rosenbaum, P., Kertoy, M., Petrenchik, T. (2006). Predictors of the leisure and recreation participation of children with physical disabilities: A structural equation modeling analysis. *Child. Health Care, 35*(3), 209-234.
[http://dx.doi.org/10.1207/s15326888chc3503_2]

Lehnhard, G., Manta, S., Palma, L. (2012). A prática de atividade física na história de vida de pessoas com deficiência física. *Rev. Educ. Fis. UEM, 23*(1), 45-56.
[http://dx.doi.org/10.4025/reveducfis.v23i1.13795]

Lollar, D.J. (2002). Public health and disability: Emerging opportunities. *Public Health Rep., 117*(2), 131-136.
[http://dx.doi.org/10.1016/S0033-3549(04)50119-X] [PMID: 12356997]

Maher, C.A., Williams, M.T., Olds, T., Lane, A.E. (2007). Physical and sedentary activity in adolescents with cerebral palsy. *Dev. Med. Child Neurol., 49*(6), 450-457.
[http://dx.doi.org/10.1111/j.1469-8749.2007.00450.x] [PMID: 17518932]

Malheiro, M. (2005). Integração/inclusão de jovens com spina bífida no ensino regular. *Revista de Educação*

Especial e Reabilitação, 12(1-2), 35-47.

Malina, R.M., Little, B.B. (2008). Physical activity: The present in the context of the past. *Am. J. Hum. Biol., 20*(4), 373-391.
[http://dx.doi.org/10.1002/ajhb.20772] [PMID: 18433002]

Marques, A., Diniz, J., Costa, F., Contramestre, J., Piéron, M. (2009). Percepção de saúde, competência e imagem corporal dos alunos que frequentam os estabelecimentos militares de ensino em Portugal. *Boletim SPEF, 34*, 51-63.

Marques, A., Maldonado, I., Peralta, M., Santos, S. (2015). Exploring psychosocial correlates of physical activity among children and adolescents with spina bifida. *Disabil. Health J., 8*(1), 123-129. a
[http://dx.doi.org/10.1016/j.dhjo.2014.06.008] [PMID: 25091554]

Marques, A., Martins, J., Peralta, M., Catunda, R., Nunes, L.S. (2016). European adults' physical activity socio-demographic correlates: A cross-sectional study from the European Social Survey. *PeerJ, 4*, e2066.
[http://dx.doi.org/10.7717/peerj.2066] [PMID: 27280072]

Marques, A., Sarmento, H., Martins, J., Saboga Nunes, L. (2015). Prevalence of physical activity in European adults - Compliance with the World Health Organization's physical activity guidelines. *Prev. Med., 81*, 333-338. b
[http://dx.doi.org/10.1016/j.ypmed.2015.09.018] [PMID: 26449407]

Matos, M., Simões, C., Tomé, G., Camacho, I., Ferreira, M., Ramiro, L. Equipa Aventura Social. (2012). A saúde dos adolescentes portugueses: Relatório do estudo HBSC 2010.

Martin, J.J. (2013). Benefits and barriers to physical activity for individuals with disabilities: A social-relational model of disability perspective. *Disabil. Rehabil., 35*(24), 2030-2037.
[http://dx.doi.org/10.3109/09638288.2013.802377] [PMID: 23781907]

Mauerberg de Castro, E. (2005). *Atividade Física Adaptada.* Ribeirão Preto, SP: Tecmedd, Murphy, N., Carbone, P., & Council on Children With Disabilities (2008). Promoting the participation of children with disabilities in sports, recreation, and physical activities. *Pediatrics, 121*(5), 1057-1061.
[http://dx.doi.org/10.1542/peds.2008-0566]

Neter, J.E., Schokker, D.F., de Jong, E., Renders, C.M., Seidell, J.C., Visscher, T.L. (2011). The prevalence of overweight and obesity and its determinants in children with and without disabilities. *J. Pediatr., 158*(5), 735-739.
[http://dx.doi.org/10.1016/j.jpeds.2010.10.039] [PMID: 21146183]

Ng, S.W., Popkin, B.M. (2012). Time use and physical activity: A shift away from movement across the globe. *Obes. Rev., 13*(8), 659-680.
[http://dx.doi.org/10.1111/j.1467-789X.2011.00982.x] [PMID: 22694051]

Othero, M., Dalmaso, A. (2009). Pessoas com deficiência na atenção primária: Discurso e prática de profissionais em um centro de saúde-escola *Interface: Comunicação, Saúde, Educação, Botucatu, 13*(28), 177-188.
[http://dx.doi.org/1590/ S1414-32832009000100015]

Pate, R.R., Davis, M.G., Robinson, T.N., Stone, E.J., McKenzie, T.L., Young, J.C. (2006). Promoting physical activity in children and youth: A leadership role for schools: A scientific statement from the American Heart Association Council on Nutrition, Physical Activity, and Metabolism (Physical Activity Committee) in collaboration with the Councils on Cardiovascular Disease in the Young and Cardiovascular Nursing. *Circulation, 114*(11), 1214-1224.
[http://dx.doi.org/10.1161/CIRCULATIONAHA.106.177052] [PMID: 16908770]

Perrier, M.J., Shirazipour, C.H., Latimer-Cheung, A.E. (2015). Sport participation among individuals with acquired physical disabilities: Group differences on demographic, disability, and Health Action Process Approach constructs. *Disabil. Health J., 8*(2), 216-222.
[http://dx.doi.org/10.1016/j.dhjo.2014.09.009] [PMID: 25458978]

Pijl, S., Frostad, P. (2010). Peer Acceptance and Self-Concept of Students with Disabilities in Regular

Education. *Eur. J. Spec. Needs Educ.,* *25*(1), 93-105.
[http://dx.doi.org/10.1080/08856250903450947]

Pitanga, F. (2002). Epidemiologia, atividade física e saúde. *Revista Brasileira de Ciência e Movimento,* *10*(3), 49-54.

Riley, B.B., Rimmer, J.H., Wang, E., Schiller, W.J. (2008). A conceptual framework for improving the accessibility of fitness and recreation facilities for people with disabilities. *J. Phys. Act. Health,* *5*(1), 158-168.
[http://dx.doi.org/10.1123/jpah.5.1.158] [PMID: 18209261]

Rimmer, J.H., Chen, M.D., McCubbin, J.A., Drum, C., Peterson, J. (2010). Exercise intervention research on persons with disabilities: What we know and where we need to go. *Am. J. Phys. Med. Rehabil.,* *89*(3), 249-263.
[http://dx.doi.org/10.1097/PHM.0b013e3181c9fa9d] [PMID: 20068432]

Rimmer, J.H., Riley, B., Wang, E., Rauworth, A., Jurkowski, J. (2004). Physical activity participation among persons with disabilities: Barriers and facilitators. *Am. J. Prev. Med.,* *26*(5), 419-425.
[http://dx.doi.org/10.1016/j.amepre.2004.02.002] [PMID: 15165658]

Rimmer, J.A., Rowland, J.L. (2008). Physical activity for youth with disabilities: A critical need in an underserved population. *Dev. Neurorehabil.,* *11*(2), 141-148.
[http://dx.doi.org/10.1080/17518420701688649] [PMID: 18415819]

Roberts, K., Cavill, N., Hancock, C., Rutter, H. (2013). *Social and Economic Inequalities in Diet and Physical Activity.* London: Public Health England.

Rodrigues, D. (2005). Corporeidade e Exclusão Social. In CDI-FMH (Ed.), *O corpo que (des)conhecemos* Cruz Quebrada: Faculdade de Motricidade Humana.

Roult, R., Carbonneau, H., Chan, T., Belley-Ranger, E., Duquette, M. (2014). Physical activity and the development of the built environment in schools for youth with a functional disability in Quebec. *Sport Sci. Rev.,* *23*(5-6), 225-240.
[http://dx.doi.org/10.1515/ssr-2015-0003]

Rowe, D.A., Raedeke, T.D., Wiersma, L.D., Mahar, M.T. (2007). Investigating the youth physical activity promotion model: Internal structure and external validity evidence for a potential measurement model. *Pediatr. Exerc. Sci.,* *19*(4), 420-435.
[http://dx.doi.org/10.1123/pes.19.4.420] [PMID: 18089909]

Safania, A., Mokhtari, R. (2012). Participation in sports activities in leisure time and quality of life of active and inactive disabled war veterans and disabled people. *Int. Res. J. Appl. Basic Sci.,* *3*(4), 859-867.
[http://dx.doi.org/10.1016/j.archger.2017.07.025]

Sallis, J.F., Prochaska, J.J., Taylor, W.C. (2000). A review of correlates of physical activity of children and adolescents. *Med. Sci. Sports Exerc.,* *32*(5), 963-975.
[http://dx.doi.org/10.1097/00005768-200005000-00014] [PMID: 10795788]

Seabra, A.F., Mendonça, D.M., Thomis, M.A., Anjos, L.A., Maia, J.A. (2008). Determinantes biológicos e sócio-culturais associados à prática de atividade física de adolescentes. *Cad. Saude Publica,* *24*(4), 721-736.
[http://dx.doi.org/10.1590/S0102-311X2008000400002] [PMID: 18392349]

Sérgio, M. (2005). *O auto-conceito e a percepção do suporte social dos sdolescentes com e sem deficiência motora em ensino regular.*Dissertação apresentada à Faculdade de Motricidade Humana, Universidade Técnica de Lisboa, com vista à obtenção do Grau de Mestre em Educação Especial.

Serona, B., Arruda, G., Greguol, M. (2015). Facilitadores e barreiras percebidas para a prática de atividade física por pessoas com deficiência motora. *Revista Brasileira de Ciências do Esporte,* *37*(3), 214-221.
[http://dx.doi.org/10.1016/j.rbce.2013.09.003]

Silva, A., Duarte, E., Almeida, J. (2011). Campeonato escolar e deficiência visual: O discurso dos professores de educação física. *Movimento (ESEF/UFRGS),* *17*(2), 37-55.

[http://dx.doi.org/10.22456/1982-8918.18897]

Slater, A., Tiggemann, M. (2011). Gender differences in adolescent sport participation, teasing, self-objectification and body image concerns. *J. Adolesc., 34*(3), 455-463.
[http://dx.doi.org/10.1016/j.adolescence.2010.06.007] [PMID: 20643477]

Smith, B.J., Cheung, N.W., Bauman, A.E., Zehle, K., McLean, M. (2005). Postpartum physical activity and related psychosocial factors among women with recent gestational diabetes mellitus. *Diabetes Care, 28*(11), 2650-2654.
[http://dx.doi.org/10.2337/diacare.28.11.2650] [PMID: 16249534]

Solish, A., Perry, A., Minnes, P. (2010). Participation of Children with and without Disabilities in Social, Recreational and Leisure Activities. *J. Appl. Res. Intellect. Disabil., 23*(3), 226-236.
[http://dx.doi.org/10.1111/j.1468-3148.2009.00525.x]

United States Department of Health and Human Services [USDHHS]. *Physical Activity Guidelines Advisory Committee Scientific Report.* Washington D.C.: U.S. Department of Health and Human Services.

Van den Berghe, L., Vansteenkiste, M., Cardon, G., Kirk, D., Haerens, L. (2014). Research on selfdetermination in physical education: Key findings and proposals for future research. *Phys. Educ. Sport Pedagogy, 19*(1), 97-121.
[http://dx.doi.org/10.1080/17408989.2012.732563]

Van Der Horst, K., Paw, M.J., Twisk, J.W., Van Mechelen, W. (2007). A brief review on correlates of physical activity and sedentariness in youth. *Med. Sci. Sports Exerc., 39*(8), 1241-1250.
[http://dx.doi.org/10.1249/mss.0b013e318059bf35] [PMID: 17762356]

Valis, J., Gonzalez, M. (2017). Physical activity differences for college students with disabilities. *Disabil. Health J., 10*(1), 87-92.
[http://dx.doi.org/10.1016/j.dhjo.2016.09.003] [PMID: 27743789]

Wilhite, B., Shank, J. (2009). In praise of sport: Promoting sport participation as a mechanism of health among persons with a disability. *Disabil. Health J., 2*(3), 116-127.
[http://dx.doi.org/10.1016/j.dhjo.2009.01.002] [PMID: 21122750]

World Health Organization [WHO] . (2010). *Global Recommendations on Physical Activity for Health.* Geneva.

World Health Organization [WHO] . (2016). *Global Report on Diabetes.* World Health Organization. Geneva.

Zabriskie, R., Lundberg, N., Groff, D. (2005). Quality of Life and identity: The benefits of a community-based therapeutic recreation and adaptive sports program. *Ther. Recreation J., 39*(3), 176-191.

CHAPTER 10

Psychosocial Correlates of the Physical Activity of Children and Adolescents with Intellectual Disability or Motor Impairment

Sofia Santos[1,*], **Vera Figueiredo Serafim**[2], **Inês Maldonado**[2], **Fernando Gomes**[3], **Miguel Peralta**[4] and **Adilson Marques**[4]

[1] *Faculdade de Motricidade Humana, UIDEF – Instituto de Educação, Universidade de Lisboa, Portugal*

[2] *Faculdade de Motricidade Humana, Universidade de Lisboa, Portugal*

[3] *SpertLab, Faculdade de Motricidade Humana, Universidade de Lisboa, Portugal*

[4] *CIPER, Faculdade de Motricidade Humana, Universidade de Lisboa Faculdade de Motricidade Humana, Estrada da Costa, 1499-002 Cruz Quebrada, Portugal*

Abstract: The positive relationship between physical activity (PA) and health, healthy lifestyle and regular PA engagement has been pointed out in the literature. However, a significant proportion of the world's population does not engage in enough PA, and in Portugal, the situation is getting worst in terms of children and adolescents with disabilities. These subgroups tend to be inactive, facing numerous health problems and limitations in their daily lives, with consequences in their functionality and quality of life. Most of the research studies within the framework of disability are based on adults and are not specific to a kind of disability. The goal of this study is to analyse and compare the psychosocial correlates of PA of 91 children and adolescents, between 10 and 17 years, in regular schools. Of all the participants, 30 had intellectual disability (13.43±2.28), 31 (13.4±0.1) had spina bifida and 30 had (12.70±1.15) typical development. A questionnaire was applied to characterize the engagement in PA by these children, to determine their impact factors. There were significant differences in the formal and informal PA engagement of students and their parents and peers. Students with a disability tend to be less engaged both in formal and informal physical activity, however, the attitude towards PA and physical education was identical in all the students, as well as competence and health perception. Scholarly sports seem to be a good strategy for the participation of all the students in physical activities. There should be an emphasis on studying and finding solutions and strategies to enable children to have access to physical activity in and out of school.

Keywords: Competence Perception, Health Perception, Intellectual Disability, Motor Disability, Physical Activity, Psychosocial Correlates, Physical Education,

---
* **Corresponding author Sofia Santos:** Faculdade de Motricidade Humana, UIDEF – Instituto de Educação, Universidade de Lisboa, Portugal; Tel: +351214149243; E-mail: sofiasantos@fmh.ulisboa.pt

Samuel Honório, Marco Batista, Helena Mesquita & Jaime Ribeiro (Eds.)

Significant Peers, Significant Adults, Scholar Sport.

INTRODUCTION

Regular physical activity (PA) has a positive impact on health and is a key factor of healthy lifestyles (Marques, 2010), contributing to the functionality and quality of life (Visscher, Vjuik, Hartman & Scherder, 2010). People with disabilities have more co-morbidities and require extra care from health promotion and prevention services, as compared to the general population (Yen, Lin, Loh, Shi & Shu, 2009). They also present higher levels of sedentary behaviour and physical inactivity, a greater prevalence of unhealthy lifestyles, and reduced participation in community life (Hutzler & Korsensky, 2010).

Nowadays, intellectual disability is no longer defined solely based on the low intelligence quotient, but it relys on the concomitance of significant intellectual and adaptive limitations during the developmental period (American Psychiatric Association, [APA], 2013) or until adulthood (Schalock *et al.*, 2010). Motor disability is characterized by motor impairments caused by injuries in body structures responsible for movement that affect daily functioning and social participation (World Health Organization, 2001). Spina bifida is a motor disability that results from the non-closure of the neural tube (Durstine *et al.*, 2000), with an impact on daily life. According to recent conceptual models of human functioning, disability is conceptualized as the quality of the relationship between the individual and the environmental demands, emphasizing the provision of support for effective participation, instead of individual limitations (Santos, Lebre & Pereira, 2018).

In the last decade, research was mainly focused on intellectual (Schalock *et al.*, 2010) and motor (Marques *et al.*, 2015) disabilities, paediatrics and rehabilitation (Fragala-Pinkman, O'Neill, Bjornson & Boyd, 2012), PA participation (Van der Horst, Paw, Twisk & Mechelen, 2007) and PA impact on public health (Johnson, 2009; Rimmer & Rowland, 2008). Now, the focus is on education, disease prevention and health promotion through PA participation (Fragala-Pinkman *et al.*, 2012).

Even though participation in regular PA improves health, a significant part of the population does not practice enough PA to achieve its benefits (Marques, Sarmento, Martins, & Saboga Nunes, 2015). Additionally, people with intellectual disabilities are even less engaged in PA than the general population (Perrier, Shirazipour & Latimer-Cheung, 2015), justifying the need for adapted and personalized plans and programs. Besides the scarcity of evidence in this population (Patrick *et al.*, 2012; Rimmer, Chen, McCubbin, Drum & Peterson,

2010), PA engagement is known to be influenced by age, gender, type of diagnosis and other demographical variables.

Regarding the physical fitness of people with disabilities, although it may be difficult to establish due to the limitations imposed by the diagnosis information (Patrick, Sami & Dirk, 2012), it is usually lower than that of their peers without disabilities (Bodde & Seo, 2009). Notwithstanding, motor proficiency, PA level and community participation are important outcomes related to the functional status of people with disabilities (McDonald, 2002). Given this scenario, it is urgent to promote PA participation in youth, particularly in children and adolescents with disabilities (Fragala-Pinkman *et al.*, 2005).

Childhood, Adolescence & Physical Activity

Childhood and adolescence are two critical periods in human development, as competences, knowledge, attitudes and behaviours acquired in these stages are transferred into adult life (Rimmer & Rowland, 2008). Martin & Choy (2009), highlighting the importance of the development of a healthy and active lifestyle in childhood and its benefits in adult life (Lehnhard, Manta, & Palma, 2012).

The benefits of regular participation in PA on both physiological (USDHHS, 2018) and psychological (Rimmer & Rowland, 2008) levels are well documented. Exercise has been pointed out as beneficial for improvements in strength and cardiovascular capacity (Draheim, 2006), secondary conditions' prevention (contractures, spasticity decrease, fractures decrease – Oriel, George & Blatt, 2008), self-concept, perception of competence and interpersonal relations (Specht, King, Brown & Foris, 2002). However, PA levels are decreasing (Patrick *et al.*, 2012) and participation in PA tends to decline with age (Frey, Stanish & Temple, 2008). Worryingly, among children and adolescents with a disability, who tend to be less active and have lower fitness levels than their peers, this decrease is even higher (Bodde & Seo, 2009; Patrick *et al.*, 2012).

Children and adolescents with disabilities tend to engage in more sedentary activities, which require less effort, and are focused essentially on socialization (Hands & Larkin, 2006). Additionally, most of these children and adolescents do not have positive PA experiences that could lead them to become more physically active. The lack of PA in this population may compromise short and long-term health and well-being (Ferreira *et al.*, 2006). Individuals with a motor disability, who are actively and regularly engaged in PA, have better health, as well as a higher level of community participation (Crawford, Hollingsworth, Morgan & Gray, 2008). Martin & Choy (2009) suggested that being inactive increases the negative effects of having a disability.

Children with a disability tend to be weaker and more fatigue susceptible, due to higher metabolic, cardiorespiratory and mobility costs (Durstine *et al.*, 2000). An inactive lifestyle (Murphy & Carbone, 2008), as well as a busy lifestyle, bad nutritional habits, parents' emotional and financial exhaustion from therapies (Yazdani, Yee & Chung, 2013), overprotection (Martin & Choy, 2009), having less opportunities and the non-consideration of individual perceptions and preferences are some of the barriers that should be considered when promoting healthy lifestyles in schools.

Children with a motor disability tend to have higher body mass indexes and less strength and cardiorespiratory fitness than their peers without disabilities (Hands & Larkin, 2006). Similarly, children and adolescents with intellectual disabilities have lower oxygen consumption capacity, reduced cardiac response and less muscle strength (Patrick *et al.*, 2012). Among this population, having a higher risk of cardiovascular and respiratory diseases, hypertension and diabetes, gait problems, fine and gross motor skills limitations and obesity are some of the reported issues related to physical inactivity (Hutzler & Korsensky, 2010). Bryl, Matuszak & Hoffman (2013) highlighted the comorbidities associated with intellectual disability, indicating the lack of understanding of PA participation in this population. This fact associated with stigma and lower social expectations seems to reduce the relevance of PA for healthy development (*e.g.* PA as therapeutic *vs.* social participation *vs.* recreational *vs.* competition sports engagement, *etc.*) and social participation (White, Gonda, Peterson & Drum, 2011).

The lack of PA opportunities, insufficient teachers training (Murphy & Carbone, 2008; Rimmer & Rowland, 2008), fear of competition, low resistance to frustration, and parents' inactivity are some of the factors that influence the future lifestyle of children with disabilities (Rimmer & Rowland, 2008). However, the only variable with a positive association with PA engagement is participation in physical education classes and scholar sport (Van der Horst *et al.*, 2007).

Psychosocial Correlates of Physical Activity

PA determinants are complex and involve the analysis of several variables (Strauss, Rodzilsky, Burack & Colin, 2001). Correlates are defined as the set of causal factors that influence the participation (Van Der Horst *et al.*, 2007) and can be demographic, biological (*e.g.*: age, *etc.*...), psychological (*e.g.*: motivation, body awareness), behavioural (*e.g.*: sedentary vs sport participation), non-modifiable or modifiable. Some known correlates of PA levels are related to previous PA participation, encompassing social (parents' and peers' influence.) and environmental factors (*e.g.* accessibility - Van Der Horst *et al.*, 2007). Sallis,

Taylor, Dowda, Freedson & Pate (2000) studied the perception of competence, health perception, significant proxies, and accessibility/barriers.

Health perception seems to be positively related to PA participation and varies with age and gender. Knowles, Niven, Fawkner & Henretty (2009) found a decrease in PA participation of female adolescents which was not influenced by maturational level or physical characteristics, but was partially influenced by their physical perceptions. Active children and adolescents, between 12 and 17 years, had a better health perception (Spink *et al.*, 2005). Time spent in treatments and therapies does not promote a good health perception, which may influence PA participation. Children and adolescents with higher health and competence' perceptions tend to engage regularly in PA (Rowe, Raedeke, Wiersma & Mahar, 2007). Ildefonso & Simões (2008) measured the self-concept of 494 students with disabilities in which 36% reported a health problem, 15.8% reported that the problem affected their scholar life, and 18.8%, that the problem affected their daily life activities and 47.8% reported that the problem affected their social participation with peers.

Perception of competence measures the personal efficacy level of one's own abilities to perform specific tasks and is a determinant in identity construction, behavioral patternsand in the promotion of physical and psychological wellbeing (Ferreira *et al.*, 2006). Although motor proficiency is not a predictor of PA participation and perception of competence during childhood, it is very important in adolescence, increasing the commitment for PA (Barnett, Morgan, Beurden & Beard, 2008) and an active lifestyle across the life span.

The existence of a disability influences the individual and the family with a sense of incapacity, and thus the promotion of competence and efficacy is essential. The role of self-perception becomes relevant at psychological, socioemotional and capacitation levels (Paiva, Kuei, Nacif & Júnior, 2013). Parents' and peers' influence seems to be relevant to build the perception of competence (Marques, 2010). Males tend to present better perception of competence, therefore, research should focus on physical literacy in females and less active population subgroups, such as persons with disabilities (Inchley *et al.*, 2011).

Family is one of the main supports of community participation in children with disabilities (Sérgio, 2005) that might act as a barrier or facilitator for PA participation and healthy lifestyles. Parents of children with disabilities tend to overprotect them, thus preventing and sometimes avoiding their participation in competitive activities with the fear of failure or verbal abuse by other children (Rimmer & Rowland, 2008). Parents, as significant adults, influence PA participation (Marques, 2010): 31.7% of the participants reported that their parents influenced their initial engagement in PA, although they were not decisive in the involvement in activities, and only 4.1% mentioned the importance of physical education teachers. Research in this area is still scarce.

Peers' influence, especially in children and adolescents with typical development, seems to contribute to pleasure in PA engagement (Sallis *et al.*, 2002). The relationship between disability level, disability self-perception and interaction with typical peers may restrict the attitudes and behaviors of adolescents with disabilities (Sérgio, 2005). Although personal relations with typical peers are promoted in schools, Pijl, Frostad & Flem (2008) found that 25% of the students with disabilities were not well accepted by their peers, did not have many friends and did not participate in class group activities. Students with disabilities are more vulnerable to isolation and tend to establish interpersonal relations with their peers with disabilities. Therefore, it is urgent to understand the peers' influence in PA participation of children with disabilities and how this relation can promote enough practice.

Even with the increasing research on the participation of people with disabilities in PA, most studies involve adults (Peterson, Janz & Lowe, 2008). Therefore, it seems fundamental to identify and understand which factors promote PA participation among children and adolescents with different types of disabilities. The inactivity rates of people with disabilities are high, thus one of the future challenges is to design, implement and monitor specific strategies and programs for these subgroups (Marques *et al.*, 2015). The goal of this chapter is to compare PA participation of children and adolescents with and without intellectual disabilities and examine the PA psychosocial correlates of children with spina bifida.

METHODS

Sample

The total sample comprised 121 students, aged between 10 and 17 years, attending regular school. From this sample, 30 participants, 16 males and 14 females, had a previous diagnosis of a intellectual disability (13.43±2.28 years), 29 students had typical development (12.70±1.15 years) without any kind of diagnosis, and 31 students (13.4±0.1 years), 16 males and 15 females, had spina bifida. Students with intellectual disabilities were recruited randomly by their special education teachers according to the inclusion criteria. Students without a disability attending the same scholar year were also randomly selected. In order to participate in the study, the participants had to be able to fully understand and answer the questionnaire.

Procedures

Ethical approval was firstly sought and given by the Ethics Committee and the National Commission of Data Protection. Then, permission was sought from the General Directorate of Education and after its authorization, contacts were established with the directors of different schoolsto conduct the study. An informed consent explaining the study procedures was obtained by the participants and their legal guardians to grant participation in the study. Confidentiality and anonymity were guaranteed. Students from 5 schools were participated in the study.

Data was collected through questionnaire. The questionnaires were conducted in physical education classes with the help of the respective teachers. The main researcher was present when the questionnaires were being filled. Before filling the questionnaire, a researcher explained the study and was available for clarifying eventual doubts. All the students answered the same questions. Each questionnaire took about 30 minutes to be completed.

Instrument

One questionnaire comprising several items regarding PA, sociodemographic and psychosocial variables was used. The questionnaire was previously validated among children and adolescents with typical development (Marques, 2010). It involved 26 items, including identification (coded); type and importance of leisure time activities and daily routine; nutritional habits; physical and sport activities engagement; health perception and perception of competence; attitudes towards school, physical education and PA; peers and parents lifestyles; goal and tasks orientation and other sociodemographic information.

To measure PA participation, items about organized (formal) and non-organized (informal) PA and participation in physical education activities of scholar sport were asked. Attitude towards school, physical education and PA were assessed through the following questions: "what do you think about school?", "what do you think about physical education classes?" and "what do you think about regular PA participation?". Answers were given on a Likert-scale ranging from 1 ("don't like at all") to 5 ("I really like"). Five items measured the perception of competence on a 5-points Likert scale and health perception on a 4-points Likert scale (1 = "not having good health" to 4 = "Very good health". Twelve questions measured goal and task orientation and the answers ranged from 1 (no importance) to 4 (very important). To measure parents' PA participation, the students were asked: "Does your father engage in PA?" and "Does your mother do sports?". Likert-scale answers were as follows, 1-"Never"; 2- "Rarely"; 3- "At least once a week"; 4- "Don't know". The answers were then grouped into "yes, engage" or "no, do not engage". Peers' PA participation was measured by two items: the first aimed to know if the participants engaged in PA regularly with friends through a 5-points Likert-scale ranging from 1 (never) to 5 (always); while in the second, students were asked if their friends were actively engaged in PA and the answers varied from 1 (never) to 5 (daily).

Statistical Analysis

A descriptive analysis was performed for all the variables. For the comparative study between children and adolescents with and without intellectual disabilities, two tests were used: for nominal variables, the Qui-Square test was performed and ordinal (quantitative) variables were analysed using the Mann-Whitney test due to the non-normal distribution scores obtained by Shapiro-Wilk and Kolmogorov-Smirnoff tests. Data analysis was performed using the software SPSS (Statistical Package for the Social Sciences) version 21.

RESULTS

When comparing students with and without intellectual disabilities with respect to their attitude towards physical activity and physical education, the findings were similar without significant differences between groups. The mean scores of students with typical development were higher, as expected. Similar conclusions were found for the perception of competence and health perception. 74.2% of the students with spina bifida reported that they practiced PA less than 3 hours per week. Most parents (fathers and mothers) did not practice PA. Although 36.7% of the participants with spina bifida considered their friends active, 71% reported that usually, they did not engage in physical activities with friends. Only 12 students with spina bifida were engaged in both organized and non-organized PA. The findings showed no significant differences between students with spina bifida who participated in PA as compared to those who were not involved in such activity, except in perception of competence in non-organized activities, which was higher. Furthermore, there was no relationship between the types of PA and psychosocial correlates. The results are presented in Table **1**.

Table 1. Psychosocial correlation results of students with spina bifida and students with and without intellectual disability.

	Students with ID M±SD or %	Students without ID M±SD or %	p^a	Students with spina bifida M±SD or %
Ego orientation	2.73±.54	2.67±.60	.83	3.0±.6
Task orientation	1.73±.47	1.60±.39	.20	3.1±.4
Attitude towards PA	4.15±.97	4.41±1.12	.11	3.9±1.0

(Table 1) cont.....

	Students with ID M±SD or %	Students without ID M±SD or %	p^a	Students with spina bifida M±SD or %
Attitude towards PE	3.86±.99	4.07±1.07	.33	3.73±1.3
Perception of competence	3.45±1.01	3.96±.81	.04	3.1±.8
Health perception	3.07±.98	3.38±.73	.25	2.6±1.0
School sport			.78	
Yes	30.0%	33.3%		19.4%
No	70.0%	66.7%		80.6%
Fathers' PA			.01	
No	75.0%	37.9%		82.2%
Yes	25.0%	62.1%		17.9%
Mother's PA			.02	
No	62.5%	31.0%		82.2%
Yes	37.5%	69.0%		17.9%
PA with peers	2.10±1.24	3.30±1.32	.001	2.1±1
Informal PA frequency	2.25±1.48	3.93±1.6	<.001	---
Formal PA frequency	2.55±1.79	3.43±1.63	.004	---
PA time per week: Less than 3h per week More than 3h per week	92.9% 7.1%	65.5% 34.5%	.012	74.2% 25.8%

M, mean; SD, standard deviation; ID, intellectual disabilities; PA, physical activity; PE, physical education
[a]For the difference between students with ID and without ID.

School gives opportunities to all students, with and without disabilities, to engage in PA, both in physical education classes and school sports. However, only 9 students with intellectual disabilities, 6 students with spina bifida and 10 students without a disability participated in school sports. Students without disabilities tend to present, as expected, higher mean scores in all the variables. There are significant differences in PA participation of parents of children with intellectual disabilities who tend to be more inactive than their peers. This finding was similar to the parents of students with spina bifida. Only 6 fathers and 9 mothers of students with intellectual disabilities and 5 fathers and 5 mothers of students with spina bifida were physically active. Whereas, parents of the participants with typical development participated in PA ($N_{fathers} = 18$; $N_{mothers}=20$). In general, students with a disability tend to be less engaged in PA than their peers without a disability.

DISCUSSION

The goal of this article was to compare the psychosocial correlates of PA participation between children and adolescents with and without an intellectual disability and to analyse the same correlates for students with spina bifida. Overall, there are significant differences in formal and informal PA participation of students, their parents and peers. Students with a disability tend to be less engaged both in formal and informal physical activity (Temple *et al.*, 2006). The attitude towards PA and physical education seems to be identical between all the students, as well as the perception of competence and health perception, which was not expected. School sports seems a good strategy for promoting students' participation in PA, as no significant differences between participants were observed.

According to Rimmer *et al.*, (2004) individuals with a disability did not have active routines and active lifestyles. Patrick *et al.* (2012) remind that promoting PA levels must be an immediate goal for promoting wellbeing and healthy lifestyles among this population. Therefore, the availability of PA opportunities in schools should be increased, due to its importance for social participation in childhood and adolescence, and for PA engagement in adult life (Murphy & Carbone, 2008; Rimmer & Rowland, 2008). The increase in teacher's knowledge about exercise prescription for groups with disabilities should also be considered (Durstine *et al.*, 2000). PA can even act as a rehabilitation method (Yen *et al.*, 2012), complementing other therapeutic interventions (Bryl *et al.*, 2013).

Ego and task orientation are influenced by motivation for task performance. The first one is more associated with external benefits and personal outcomes (*e.g.*: social status - Duda, 1989). On the other hand, task orientation emphasizes the skill proficiency, its empowerment, cooperation and socialization, leading to better self-esteem and a healthier lifestyle. Therefore, task orientation seems to be essential for PA engagement (Papaioannou, Bebetsos, Theodorakis, Christodoulidis, & Kouli, 2006), but both the correlates complement each other (Fox, Goudas, Biddle, Duda, & Armstrong, 1994). The results of both the variables did not show significant differences between participants. The findings point out that children and adolescents with intellectual disabilities present higher scores in ego orientation rather than in task orientation. Children with a disability tend to show lower resistance to frustration as well as lower motivation and concentration in tasks (Harris, 2006).

Our findings did not present any significant differences in the attitude of students with and without disabilities towards PA, which was not expected. A positive relationship between health/perception of competence and PA participation is evidenced in the literature (Marques *et al.*, 2009); a healthy student with a positive perception of competence tends to present a more positive attitude towards PA. Health perception presents the same positive relation with PA, varying with age and gender (Ildefonso & Simões, 2008; Knowles *et al.*, 2009). The differences in health competence and perception of competence were not significant, although the mean scores of students without a disability were higher. The relation between PA and health perception was not significant. It is possible to infer that in students with spina bifida, time spent in therapeutic intervention and treatments does not promote health perception.

Perception of competence related to motor proficiency in childhood and adolescence may act as a facilitator for PA participation in adult life (Barnett *et al.*, 208). A motivated child tends to participate more and feel more competent. The negative attitudes of stigma and devaluation (Santos & Franco, 2017) restraint from building a positive social identity, resulting in a lower perception of competence in individuals with disabilities. The perception of competence of the participants with spina bifida is related to informal PA (Marques *et al.*, 2015). There is still a lack of evidence in this specific subgroup.

Parents' and peers' influence is a key point in the development of perception of competence (Martin & Choy, 2009) and as expected, participation in PA with peers is higher among students without a disability. The findings showed no difference between PA engagement and peers' influence. 70% of the participants stated that they rarely or never engage in PA with their peers, even in the school. This is an issue to consider in the future because the interaction with typical peers seems to be a motivational strategy for promoting PA in this population (Stanisic, 2012). Nevertheless, more studies are needed. Martin (2006) reported that although there is a relationship between PA participation and parents/peer's motivation, the pleasure and satisfaction gained by PA seems to be a significant correlate among adolescents with spina bifida.

The non-participation in PA of parents, especially in the case of students with a disability, tends to act as a barrier to their children's PA participation (Yazdani *et al.*, 2013). Parents tend to give more opportunities for practicing PA when they are aware of its benefits (Johnson, 2009). According to our findings, children whose parents engage in PA at least 3 hours per week tend to be more active (Yazdani *et al.*, 2013); however, further studies are needed. Overall, parents of children with a disability do not engage regularly in PA. The limitations in matching professional activity with PA, associated with less active habits and increased cost of other therapeutic services and supports, tend to restrain PA participation of children with disabilities. These adults may have a significant role in PA promotion (Yazdani *et al.*, 2013).

Participation in school sport seems to be a winning strategy for the promotion of healthy lifestyles, allowing students, with and without a disability, to be physically engaged (Frey *et al.*, 2008) in a structured and regular PA (Marques, 2010) and to interact with typical peers *vs.* special classes (Menear, 2007). The preference by organized and formal activities was also reported by Minnes, Burbidge & Abells (2008). Students without a disability tend to present higher mean scores in formal PA participation (Frey *et al.* 2008). PA frequency presents significant differences between students with and without disabilities.

The reduced and restricted geographical sample is one limitation of this study. Therefore, it is suggested that future studies have significant and representative samples for an overview of national PA participation in order to identify barriers and facilitators for healthy lifestyles promotion. PA-specific programs' design (frequency, intensity, quantity and type of exercise) and monitoring are still lacking in our country. One of the strengths of this study that should be emphasized is the opportunity for children and adolescents (with and without disability) to speak for themselves and to give their self-perception.

CONCLUDING REMARKS

Physical inactivity in paediatric ages is a significant predictor of physical inactivity in adult life (Lehnhard *et al.*, 2012), which arouses the need to identify strategies that successfully promote social participation and regular PA engagement of children and adolescents with disabilities. Findings show the relevance of health perception and perception of competence, as well as significant adults' and peers' impact on such engagement. Furthermore, recent educational legislation states that all the students, with and without disabilities, should participate in the schoolactivities . This inclusion will demand a change in theory and practice, and physical education and school sports can assume an important role in this process (Aguiar & Duarte, 2005). Nevertheless, PA-specific and adapted programs for these children are still scarce, therefore, research in this area should be promoted.

CONSENT FOR PUBLICATION

Not applicable.

CONFLICT OF INTEREST

The author confirms that this chapter contents have no conflict of interest.

ACKNOWLEDGEMENTS

Declared none.

REFERENCES

Aguiar, J., Duarte, E. (2005). Educação Inclusiva: um estudo na área da Educação Física. *Rev. Bras. Educ. Espec., 11*(2), 223-240.
[http://dx.doi.org/10.1590/S1413-65382005000200005]

American Psychiatric Association. (2013). *Diagnostic and Statistical Manual of Mental Disorders – DSM5™.* (5th ed.). Arlington, VA: American Psychiatric Association.

Barnett, L.M., Morgan, P.J., van Beurden, E., Beard, J.R. (2008). Perceived sports competence mediates the relationship between childhood motor skill proficiency and adolescent physical activity and fitness: a longitudinal assessment. *Int. J. Behav. Nutr. Phys. Act., 5*(40), 40.
[http://dx.doi.org/10.1186/1479-5868-5-40] [PMID: 18687148]

Bodde, A.E., Seo, D-C. (2009). A review of social and environmental barriers to physical activity for adults with intellectual disabilities. *Disabil. Health J., 2*(2), 57-66.
[http://dx.doi.org/10.1016/j.dhjo.2008.11.004] [PMID: 21122744]

Bryl, W., Matuszak, K., Hoffmann, K. (2013). Physical Activity of children and adolescents with intellectual disabilities - a public health problem. *Hygeia Public Health., 48*(1), 1-5.

Crawford, A., Hollingsworth, H.H., Morgan, K., Gray, D.B. (2008). People with mobility impairments: Physical activity and quality of participation. *Disabil. Health J., 1*(1), 7-13.
[http://dx.doi.org/10.1016/j.dhjo.2007.11.004] [PMID: 21122706]

Draheim, C.C. (2006). Cardiovascular disease prevalence and risk factors of persons with mental retardation. *Ment. Retard. Dev. Disabil. Res. Rev., 12*(1), 3-12.
[http://dx.doi.org/10.1002/mrdd.20095] [PMID: 16435328]

Duda, J. (1989). Relashionship between task and ego orientation and the perceived purpose of sport among high school athletes. *J. Sports Exer., 11*(3), 318-335.
[http://dx.doi.org/10.1123/jsep.11.3.318]

Durstine, L., Painter, P., Franklin, B., Morgan, D., Pitetti, K., Roberts, S. (2000). Physycal activity for the chronically ill and disabled. *Sports Med., 30*(3), 207-219.
[http://dx.doi.org/0112-1642/00/0009-0207]

Ferreira, I., van der Horst, K., Wendel-Vos, W., Kremers, S., van Lenthe, F.J., Brug, J. (2007). Environmental correlates of physical activity in youth - a review and update. *Obes. Rev., 8*(2), 129-154.
[http://dx.doi.org/10.1111/j.1467-789X.2006.00264.x] [PMID: 17300279]

Fox, K., Goudas, M., Biddle, S., Duda, J., Armstrong, N. (1994). Children's task and ego goal profiles in sport. *Br. J. Educ. Psychol., 64*(Pt 2), 253-261.
[http://dx.doi.org/10.1111/j.2044-8279.1994.tb01100.x] [PMID: 8075016]

Fragala-Pinkham, M.A., Haley, S.M., Rabin, J., Kharasch, V.S. (2005). A fitness program for children with disabilities. *Phys. Ther., 85*(11), 1182-1200.
[http://dx.doi.org/10.1093/ptj/85.11.1182] [PMID: 16253047]

Frey, G.C., Stanish, H.I., Temple, V.A. (2008). Physical activity of youth with intellectual disability: review and research agenda. *Adapt. Phys. Activ. Q., 25*(2), 95-117.
[http://dx.doi.org/10.1123/apaq.25.2.95] [PMID: 18493087]

Harris, J. (2006). *Intellectual Disability: Understanding Its Development, Causes, Classification, Evaluation and Treatment.* Oxford University Press.

Hands, B., Larkin, D. (2006). Physical fitness differences in children with and without motor learning difficulties. *Eur. J. Spec. Needs Educ., 21*(4), 447-456.

[http://dx.doi.org/10.1080/08856250600956410]

Hutzler, Y., Korsensky, O. (2010). Motivational correlates of physical activity in persons with an intellectual disability: a systematic literature review. *J. Intellect. Disabil. Res., 54*(9), 767-786.
[http://dx.doi.org/10.1111/j.1365-2788.2010.01313.x] [PMID: 20712695]

Ildefonso, I., Simões, C. (2008). A percepção da diferença no autoconceito dos adolescentes com necessidades educativas especiais: Estudo das variáveis contextuais que influenciam a percepção da diferença na actividade e no autoconceito. *Revista de Educação Especial e Reabilitação, 15*, 65-90.

Inchley, J., Kirby, J., Currie, C. (2011). Longitudinal changes in physical self-perceptions and associations with physical activity during adolescence. *Pediatr. Exerc. Sci., 23*(2), 237-249.
[http://dx.doi.org/10.1123/pes.23.2.237] [PMID: 21633136]

Johnson, C.C. (2009). The benefits of physical activity for youth with developmental disabilities: a systematic review. *Am. J. Health Promot., 23*(3), 157-167.
[http://dx.doi.org/10.4278/ajhp.070930103] [PMID: 19149420]

Knowles, A.M., Niven, A.G., Fawkner, S.G., Henretty, J.M. (2009). A longitudinal examination of the influence of maturation on physical self-perceptions and the relationship with physical activity in early adolescent girls. *J. Adolesc., 32*(3), 555-566.
[http://dx.doi.org/10.1016/j.adolescence.2008.06.001] [PMID: 18692232]

Lehnhard, G., Manta, S., Palma, L. (2012). A Prática de atividade física na História de vida de pessoas com deficiência física. *Rev. Educ. Fis. UEM, 23*(1), 45-56.
[http://dx.doi.org/10.4025/reveducfis.v23i1.13795]

McDonald, C.M. (2002). Physical activity, health impairments, and disability in neuromuscular disease. *Am. J. Phys. Med. Rehabil., 81*(11) (Suppl.), S108-S120.
[http://dx.doi.org/10.1097/00002060-200211001-00012] [PMID: 12409816]

Martin, J.J., Choi, Y.S. (2009). Parents' physical activity-related perceptions of their children with disabilities. *Disabil. Health J., 2*(1), 9-14.
[http://dx.doi.org/10.1016/j.dhjo.2008.09.001] [PMID: 21122737]

Marques, A. (2010). *A escola, a educação física e a promoção de estilos de vida activa e saudável: Estudo de um caso.*. Dissertação apresentada à Faculdade de Motricidade Humana com vista à obtenção do grau de Doutor em Ciências da Educação. Universidade Técnica de Lisboa (documento não publicado). .

Marques, A., Maldonado, I., Peralta, M., Santos, S. (2015). Exploring psychosocial correlates of physical activity among children and adolescents with spina bifida. *Disabil. Health J., 8*(1), 123-129.
[http://dx.doi.org/10.1016/j.dhjo.2014.06.008] [PMID: 25091554]

Marques, A., Sarmento, H., Martins, J., Saboga Nunes, L. (2015). Prevalence of physical activity in European adults - Compliance with the World Health Organization's physical activity guidelines. *Prev. Med., 81*, 333-338.
[http://dx.doi.org/10.1016/j.ypmed.2015.09.018] [PMID: 26449407]

Murphy, N.A., Carbone, P.S. (2008). Promoting the participation of children with disabilities in sports, recreation, and physical activities. *Pediatrics, 121*(5), 1057-1061.
[http://dx.doi.org/10.1542/peds.2008-0566] [PMID: 18450913]

Oriel, K., George, C., Blatt, J. (2008). The impact of a community based exercise program in children and adolescents with disabilities: a pilot study. *Phys. Disabil., 27*(1), 5-20.

Paiva, L., Kuei, J., Nacif, M., Júnior, C. (2013). Avaliação das alterações gastrintestinais e consumo de suplementos nutricionais por maratonistas. *Braz. J. Sports Med., 2*(2), 17-23.

Papaioannou, A., Bebetsos, E., Theodorakis, Y., Christodoulidis, T., Kouli, O. (2006). Causal relationships of sport and exercise involvement with goal orientations, perceived competence and intrinsic motivation in physical education: a longitudinal study. *J. Sports Sci., 24*(4), 367-382.
[http://dx.doi.org/10.1080/02640410400022060] [PMID: 16492601]

Patrick, C., Sami, E., Dirk, C. (2012). Physical and Metabolic Fitness of Children and Adolescents with Intellectual Disability – how to rehabilitate? In: Uner, T. (Ed.). *Latest Findings in Intellectual and Developmental Disabilities Research.*
[http://dx.doi.org/10.5772/30185]

Perrier, M.J., Shirazipour, C.H., Latimer-Cheung, A.E. (2015). Sport participation among individuals with acquired physical disabilities: group differences on demographic, disability, and Health Action Process Approach constructs. *Disabil. Health J., 8*(2), 216-222.
[http://dx.doi.org/10.1016/j.dhjo.2014.09.009] [PMID: 25458978]

Peterson, J.J., Janz, K.F., Lowe, J.B. (2008). Physical activity among adults with intellectual disabilities living in community settings. *Prev. Med., 47*(1), 101-106.
[http://dx.doi.org/10.1016/j.ypmed.2008.01.007] [PMID: 18308385]

Pijl, S., Frostad, P. (2010). Peer acceptance and self-concept of students with disabilities in regular education. *Eur. J. Spec. Needs Educ., 25*(1), 93-105.
[http://dx.doi.org/10.1080/08856250903450947]

Rimmer, J.H., Chen, M-D., McCubbin, J.A., Drum, C., Peterson, J. (2010). Exercise intervention research on persons with disabilities: what we know and where we need to go. *Am. J. Phys. Med. Rehabil., 89*(3), 249-263.
[http://dx.doi.org/10.1097/PHM.0b013e3181c9fa9d] [PMID: 20068432]

Rimmer, J.A., Rowland, J.L. (2008). Physical activity for youth with disabilities: a critical need in an underserved population. *Dev. Neurorehabil., 11*(2), 141-148.
[http://dx.doi.org/10.1080/17518420701688649] [PMID: 18415819]

Rowe, D.A., Raedeke, T.D., Wiersma, L.D., Mahar, M.T. (2007). Investigating the youth physical activity promotion model: internal structure and external validity evidence for a potential measurement model. *Pediatr. Exerc. Sci., 19*(4), 420-435.
[http://dx.doi.org/10.1123/pes.19.4.420] [PMID: 18089909]

Sallis, J.F., Prochaska, J.J., Taylor, W.C. (2000). A review of correlates of physical activity of children and adolescents. *Med. Sci. Sports Exerc., 32*(5), 963-975.
[http://dx.doi.org/10.1097/00005768-200005000-00014] [PMID: 10795788]

Santos, S., Franco, V. (2017). As atitudes face à Dificuldade Intelectual. *Revista de Educação Especial e Reabilitação, 24*, 11-25.

Santos, S., Lebre, P., Moniz-Pereira, L. (2018). Human Functioning and Rehabilitation Research: different ways to look at the conceptual model. In F. Alves, A. Rosado, L. Moniz-Pereira & D. Araújo (edts)*Research on Human Kinetics – Multidisciplinary Perspectives (Investigação em Motricidade Humana – Perspetivas pluridisciplinares)* Edições FMH.

Schalock, R., Borthwick-Duffy, S., Bradley, V., Buntinx, W., Coulter, D., Craig, E. (2010). *Intellectual Disability – Definition, Classification, and Systems of Supports.* (11th ed.). Washington, D.C.: American Association in Intellectual and Developmental Disability.

Sérgio, M. (2005). *O auto-conceito e a percepção do suporte social dos sdolescentes com e sem deficiência motora em ensino regular.* Dissertação apresentada à Faculdade de Motricidade Humana, com vista à obtenção do Grau de Mestre em Educação Especial. Universidade Técnica de Lisboa (documento não publicado).

Specht, J., King, G., Brown, E., Foris, C. (2002). The importance of leisure in the lives of persons with congenital physical disabilities. *Am. J. Occup. Ther., 56*(4), 436-445.
[http://dx.doi.org/10.5014/ajot.56.4.436] [PMID: 12125833]

Spink, K., Chad, K., Muhajarine, N., Humbert, L., Odnokon, P., Gryba, C., Anderson, K. (2005). Intrapersonal correlates of sufficiently active youth and adolescents. *Pediatr. Exerc. Sci., 17*, 124-135.
[http://dx.doi.org/10.1123/pes.17.2.124]

Stanisic, Z. (2012). Physical and Sport Activities of Intellectually Disabled Individuals. *Acta Medica*

Medianae, 51(2), 1-5.

Strauss, R.S., Rodzilsky, D., Burack, G., Colin, M. (2001). Psychosocial correlates of physical activity in healthy children. *Arch. Pediatr. Adolesc. Med., 155*(8), 897 902.
[http://dx.doi.org/10.1001/archpedi.155.8.897] [PMID: 11483116]

USDHHS. (2018). *Physical Activity Guidelines Advisory Committee Scientific Report.* Washington, DC: U.S. Department of Health and Human Services.

Van Der Horst, K., Paw, M.J., Twisk, J.W., Van Mechelen, W. (2007). A brief review on correlates of physical activity and sedentariness in youth. *Med. Sci. Sports Exerc., 39*(8), 1241-1250.
[http://dx.doi.org/10.1249/mss.0b013e318059bf35] [PMID: 17762356]

Vuijk, P.J., Hartman, E., Scherder, E., Visscher, C. (2010). Motor performance of children with mild intellectual disability and borderline intellectual functioning. *J. Intellect. Disabil. Res., 54*(11), 955-965.
[http://dx.doi.org/10.1111/j.1365-2788.2010.01318.x] [PMID: 20854287]

White, G.W., Gonda, C., Peterson, J.J., Drum, C.E. (2011). Secondary analysis of a scoping review of health promotion interventions for persons with disabilities: Do health promotion interventions for people with mobility impairments address secondary condition reduction and increased community participation? *Disabil. Health J., 4*(2), 129-139.
[http://dx.doi.org/10.1016/j.dhjo.2010.05.002] [PMID: 21419376]

World Health Organization. (2001). *International Classification of Functioning, Disability and Health: ICF..* Geneva: WHO Publishing.

Yazdani, S., Yee, C.T., Chung, P.J. (2013). Factors predicting physical activity among children with special needs. *Prev. Chronic Dis., 10*, E119.
[http://dx.doi.org/10.5888/pcd10.120283] [PMID: 23866163]

Yen, C.F., Lin, J.D., Loh, C.H., Shi, L., Hsu, S.W. (2009). Determinants of prescription drug use by adolescents with intellectual disabilities in Taiwan. *Res. Dev. Disabil., 30*(6), 1354-1366.
[http://dx.doi.org/10.1016/j.ridd.2009.06.002] [PMID: 19577427]

SUBJECT INDEX

A

Acetylcholine 11
Actions 20, 112
  health education 112
  prophylactic 20
Active children and adolescents 170
Acute myocardial infarction (AMI) 104
Adolescence and physical activity 168
Advisable exercises for diabetes 111
Aerobic 12, 18
  dance 18
  exercise attenuates 12
Aetiologies, traumatic 33
Ageing and brain consequences 8
Alcohol consumption 107
Allergy scanner 127
Alpha-adrenergic responses 5
Alzheimer's 3, 8, 9, 10, 11, 17, 114
  dementia 114
  disease 3, 8, 9, 10, 11, 17
Analysis 33, 138
  large cohort 33
  therapeutic environment 138
Animal-Assisted 135, 136, 137, 138, 139, 140,
    142, 143, 144
  activities (AAA) 136, 137
  interventions (AAI) 137
  therapies (AAT) 135, 136, 137, 138, 139,
    140, 142, 143, 144
Anthropomorphism 139
Antibody production, anti-transglutaminase
    122
Antioxidant reserves 7
Asperger syndrome 54, 70
Association of European celiac societies
    (AOECS) 125
Associations, celiac 125
Atherosclerosis 13
Atherosclerotic cerebrovascular diseases 12
Atrial 6, 14
  fibrillation 6
  natriuretic peptide 14

Atrophy 7, 8, 11, 122
  cortical 7, 8
  hippocampal 11
  villous 122
Ayres sensory integration 94
  intervention 94

B

Baroreflex responses 7
BDNF synthesis 16
Beta-adrenergic responsiveness 7
Beta-amyloid plaques 8
Bilingualism, enhancing 60
Bioactive compounds 107
Biochemical changes 8
Biological 4, 138, 156
  degradation 4
  predisposition 138
  reinforcement 156
Biophilia hypothesis 139
Biopsies 123
  intestinal 123
Blood glucose levels 105, 110, 111
  improved postprandial 105
  measuring 111
Blood vessel elasticity 4
Bone 5, 6, 13, 19, 110, 129
  density 5, 13, 110
  mass 6, 129
  mineral density 19, 129
Bourneville-pringle syndrome 70
Brain 7, 8, 9, 11, 12, 13, 16, 28, 29, 33, 34
  consequences 8
  damage 9, 28, 29, 33
  derived neurotrophic factor (BDNF) 7, 11,
    16
  function 9
  neuroplasticity 13
  neurotrophic factors 12
  plasticity 33, 34
Brain injury 27, 28, 33, 34, 35
  acquired 28